Diversity, Equity, and Inclusion in Dermatology

Editor

SUSAN C. TAYLOR

DERMATOLOGIC CLINICS

www.derm.theclinics.com

Consulting Editor
BRUCE H. THIERS

April 2023 • Volume 41 • Number 2

ELSEVIER

1600 John F. Kennedy Boulevard • Suite 1800 • Philadelphia, Pennsylvania, 19103-2899

http://www.theclinics.com

DERMATOLOGIC CLINICS Volume 41, Number 2
April 2023 ISSN 0733-8635, ISBN-13: 978-0-323-93967-6

Editor: Stacy Eastman
Developmental Editor: Karen Justine S. Dino

Dermatologic Clinics (ISSN 0733-8635) is published quarterly by Elsevier Inc., 360 Park Avenue South, New York, NY 10010-1710. Months of publication are January, April, July, and October. Business and editorial offices: 1600 John F. Kennedy Blvd., Suite 1800, Philadelphia, PA 19103-2899. Customer service office: 11830 Westline Drive, St. Louis, MO 63146. Periodicals postage paid at New York, NY, and additional mailing offices. Subscription prices are USD 438.00 per year for US individuals, USD 899.00 per year for US institutions, USD 478.00 per year for Canadian individuals, USD 1,097.00 per year for Canadian institutions, USD 536.00 per year for international individuals, USD 1,097.00 per year for international institutions, USD 100.00 per year for US students/residents, USD 100.00 per year for Canadian students/residents, and USD 240 per year for international students/residents. International air speed delivery is included in all *Clinics* subscription prices. All prices are subject to change without notice. **POSTMASTER:** Send address changes to *Dermatologic Clinics*, Elsevier Health Sciences Division, Subscription Customer Service, 3251 Riverport Lane, Maryland Heights, MO 63043. **Customer Service: 1-800-654-2452 (U.S. and Canada); 314-447-8871 (outside U.S. and Canada). Fax: 314-447-8029. E-mail: journalscustomerservice-usa@elsevier.com (for print support); journalsonlinesupport-usa@elsevier.com (for online support).**

Reprints. For copies of 100 or more, of articles in this publication, please contact the Commercial Reprints Department, Elsevier Inc., 360 Park Avenue South, New York, New York 10010-1710. Tel.: 212-633-3874; Fax: 212-633-3820; Email: reprints@elsevier.com.

The *Dermatologic Clinics* is covered in *MEDLINE/PubMed (Index Medicus), Current Contents/Clinical Medicine, Excerpta Medica, Chemical Abstracts,* and *ISI/BIOMED.*

Contributors

CONSULTING EDITOR

BRUCE H. THIERS, MD
Professor and Chairman Emeritus, Department
of Dermatology and Dermatologic Surgery,
Medical University of South Carolina,
Charleston, South Carolina, USA

EDITOR

SUSAN C. TAYLOR, MD, FAAD
Bernett L. Johnson Endowed Professor of
Dermatology, Vice Chair for Diversity, Equity
and Inclusion, Department of Dermatology,
Perelman School of Medicine, University of
Pennsylvania, Philadelphia, Pennsylvania, USA

AUTHORS

PAMELA S. ALLEN, MD
Associate Professor and Chair, Department of
Dermatology, Carl J. Herzog Chair in
Dermatology, Director, Residency Training
Program, Founder Director, Mark Allen Everett,
MD, Skin of Color Symposium, Chair, OU
College of Medicine Diversity Alliance Task
Force, Board Member, Skin of Color Society,
University of Oklahoma College of Medicine,
Oklahoma City, Oklahoma, USA

VICTORIA BARBOSA, MD, MPH, MBA
Associate Professor, University of Chicago
Medicine Section of Dermatology, Chicago,
Illinois, USA

SACHARITHA BOWERS, MD, FAAD
Associate Professor of Dermatology, Division
of Dermatology, Department of Internal
Medicine, Loyola University Medical Center,
Stritch School of Medicine, Maywood, Illinois,
USA

STAFFORD G. BROWN III, MS
Eastern Virginia Medical School, William &
Mary Raymond A. Mason School of Business

AILEEN Y. CHANG, MD
Assistant Professor of Clinical Dermatology,
Department of Dermatology, University of
California, San Francisco, Zuckerberg San
Francisco General Hospital, San Francisco,
California, USA

CARYN B.C. COBB, BA
The Warren Alpert Medical School of Brown
University

KAMARIA COLEMAN, BS
Medical Student, Southern Illinois University
School of Medicine,Springfield, Illinois, USA

FARINOOSH DADRASS, MD, MS
Loyola University Chicago Stritch School of
Medicine, Maywood, Illinois, USA

NADA ELBULUK, MD, MSc
Department of Dermatology, Keck School of
Medicine of USC, University of Southern
California, Los Angeles, California, USA

NKANYEZI FERGUSON, MD
Department of Dermatology, University of
Missouri, Columbia, Missouri, USA

JULIA L. GAO, BD
The Fenway Institute, Fenway Health, Department of Dermatology, Beth Israel Deaconess Medical Center, Boston, Massachusetts, USA; George Washington University School of Medicine & Health Sciences, Washington, DC, USA; Dartmouth-Hitchcock Medical Center, Lebanon, New Hampshire, USA

JANE M. GRANT-KELS, MD, FAAD
Professor of Dermatology, Pathology, and Pediatrics, Vice Chair, Department of Dermatology, University of Connecticut School of Medicine, Farmington, Connecticut, USA; Adjunct Professor, Department of Dermatology, University of Florida College of Medicine, Gainesville, Florida, USA

KARINA GRULLON, BS
University of Chicago Pritzker School of Medicine

VALERIE M. HARVEY, MD, MPH
Hampton University Skin of Color Research Institute, Hampton Roads Center for Dermatology

CANDRICE HEATH, MD
Assistant Professor, Department of Dermatology, Temple University Lewis Katz School of Medicine, Philadelphia, Pennsylvania, USA

KANIKA KAMAL, BA
Harvard Medical School, Harvard University, Boston, Massachusetts, USA

HENRY W. LIM, MD
Department of Dermatology, Henry Ford Health, Detroit, Michigan, USA

BONNIE SIMPSON MASON, MD
Medical Director of Diversity, Equity, and Inclusion, American College of Surgeons, Washington, DC, USA

NATASHA M. MICKEL, PhD
Assistant Professor, Director, Multicultural Engagement, Director, Oklahoma Center for Mentoring Excellence, University of Oklahoma Health Sciences Center, Department of Family and Preventive Medicine, University of

Oklahoma College of Medicine, Office of Diversity, Inclusion, and Community Engagement, Oklahoma City, Oklahoma, USA

ANANYA MUNJAL, MS
University of Iowa Carver College of Medicine, Iowa City, Iowa, USA

JENNY E. MURASE, MD, FAAD
Department of Dermatology, University of California, San Francisco, San Francisco, California, USA; Department of Dermatology, Palo Alto Foundation Medical Group, Mountain View, California, USA

DEDEE F. MURRELL, MA, BMBCH, MD, FRCP, FACD
Department of Dermatology, St. George Hospital, University of New South Wales, Sydney, Australia

TEMITAYO A. OGUNLEYE, MD, MHCI
Perelman School of Medicine, University of Pennsylvania, Philadelphia, Pennsylvania, USA

AMIT G. PANDYA, MD
Adjunct Professor at UT Southwestern, Department of Dermatology, Palo Alto Foundation Medical Group, Sunnyvale, California, USA; Department of Dermatology, The University of Texas Southwestern Medical Center, Dallas, Texas, USA

JENNIFER PARKER, MD, PhD, MPH
Chief Dermatology Resident, Department of Dermatology, Temple University Lewis Katz School of Medicine, Philadelphia, Pennsylvania, USA

KLINT PEEBLES, MD
Department of Dermatology, Kaiser-Permanente Mid-Atlantic Permanente Medical Group, Largo, Maryland, USA

ELLEN N. PRITCHETT, MD, MPH
Department of Dermatology, Howard University College of Medicine, Washington, DC, USA

RAMIRO RODRIGUEZ, MD
Department of Internal Medicine, The University of Texas Rio Grande Valley, Weslaco, Texas, USA; Dermatology Fellow/Instructor, Department of Dermatology,

University of Colorado Anschutz Medical
Campus, Aurora, Colorado, USA

KANADE SHINKAI, MD, PhD
Department of Dermatology, University of
California, San Francisco, San Francisco,
California, USA

NICOLE C. SYDER, BA
Department of Dermatology, Keck School of
Medicine of USC, University of Southern
California, Los Angeles, California, USA

JANELL M. TULLY, BS
Department of Dermatology, University of
California, San Francisco, San Francisco,

California, USA; University of Arizona College
of Medicine Phoenix, Phoenix, Arizona, USA

REBECCA VASQUEZ, MD
Department of Dermatology, The University of
Texas Southwestern Medical Center, Dallas,
Texas, USA

MICHELLE WEIR, MD, FAAD
Assistant Professor of Clinical Dermatology,
Perelman School of Medicine, University of
Pennsylvania, Philadelphia, Pennsylvania, USA

KIYANNA WILLIAMS, MD
Department of Dermatology, Cleveland Clinic,
Cleveland, Ohio, USA

Contents

compensation persist. Herein, we review trends in gender differences among leadership positions in academic medicine with a particular focus on dermatology, evaluate the roles of mentorship, motherhood, and gender bias on gender equity, and discuss constructive solutions for addressing gender inequities that persist in academic medicine today.

The increasing diversification of the United States has led to more racially and ethnically discordant visits between health care providers and patients; this is especially true in dermatology due to the lack of diversity in the field. Diversifying the health care workforce has been shown to reduce health care disparities and is an ongoing goal of dermatology. Improving cultural competence and humility among physicians is an important part of addressing health care inequities. This article reviews cultural competence, cultural humility, and practices dermatologists can incorporate to address this challenge.

Unconscious biases (also known as implicit biases) are involuntary stereotypes or attitudes held about certain groups of people that may influence our behaviors, understandings, and actions, often with unintended detrimental consequences. Implicit bias appears in multiple facets of medical education, training, and promotion with negative effects on diversity and equity efforts. Notable health disparities exist among minority groups in the United States, which may partly be attributable to unconscious biases. Although there is little evidence supporting the effectiveness of current bias/diversity training programming, standardization and blinding may be helpful, evidence-based methods to reduce implicit bias.

Microaggressions are directed unconsciously to people of color or other minority groups, and the accumulated experience of multiple microaggressions over a lifetime have detrimental effects on mental health. In the clinical setting, both physicians and patients can commit microaggressions. Patients experiencing a microaggression from their provider suffer emotional distress and distrust resulting in decreased service utilization, reduced adherence, and poorer physical and mental health. Physicians and medical trainees, particularly those of color, women and LGBTQIA members, have increasingly experienced microaggressions committed by patients. Learning to recognize and address microaggressions in the clinical setting creates a more supportive and inclusive environment.

Dermatologists can play a key role in improving health equity for sexual and gender diverse (SGD) patients through cultivating awareness of how their patients' sexual and gender identity may affect their skin health, developing SGD-inclusive curricula and safe spaces in medical training, promoting workforce diversity, practicing with intersectionality in mind, and engaging in advocacy for their patients, whether it be through daily practice, legislative and public policy initiatives, or research.

The social determinants of health (SDoH) have significant influences on health and lead to health disparities in a variety of complex and intersecting ways. They are the nonmedical factors that must be addressed to improve health outcomes and achieve greater health equity. They are shaped by the structural determinants of health and impact individual socioeconomic status as well as the health of entire communities. Part 1 of this 2-part review aims to shed light on how the SDoH impact health and their specific implications on dermatologic health disparities.

The social determinants of health (SDoH) impact health and lead to health disparities in a variety of complex and intersecting ways. They are the nonmedical factors that must be addressed to improve health outcomes and achieve greater health equity. The SDoH contribute to dermatologic health disparities and decreasing these disparities requires multilevel action. Part 2 of this 2-part review offers a framework that dermatologists can use to help address the SDoH both at the point of care and in the health care system at large.

Health disparities are differences in health or disease incidence, prevalence, severity, or disease burden that are experienced by disadvantaged populations. Their root causes are attributed in large part to socially determined factors, including educational level of attainment, socioeconomic status, and physical and social environments. There is an expanding body of evidence documenting differences in dermatologic health status among underserved populations. In this review, the authors highlight inequities in outcomes across 5 dermatologic conditions, including psoriasis, acne, cutaneous melanoma, hidradenitis suppurativa, and atopic dermatitis.

Racial and ethnic disparities exist across a wide range of disease areas and clinical services. Becoming familiar with the history of race in America, and how it has been used to structure laws or policies that drive inequities in the social determinants of health, even today, is necessary to mitigate these disparities across medicine.

Race and racism are rooted in the man-made belief that the color of a person's skin determines a person's hierarchal rank in humanity. Early scientific theories of poly-genics and misleading scientific studies were used to promote the concept of the inferiority of people of color and to support and maintain the institution of slavery. These discriminatory practices have filtered into society as structural racism, including the field of medicine. Structural racism has led to health disparities in black and brown communities. Dismantling structural racism requires us all to become change agents at societal and institutional levels.

Clinical trials are an essential component of research for determining the safety and efficacy of treatments for medical diseases. In order for the results of clinical trials to be generalizable to diverse populations, they must include participants at ratios that are reflective of national and global populations. A significant number of derma-tology studies not only lack racial/ethnic diversity but also fail to report data on mi-nority recruitment and enrollment. Reasons for this are multifold and are discussed in this review. Although steps have been implemented to improve this issue, greater efforts are needed for sustained and meaningful change.

Over the past few years, there have been concerted efforts to increase diversity in the field of dermatology. This has been achieved through the creation of Diversity, Equity, and Inclusion (DEI) initiatives in dermatology organizations that strive to pro-vide resources and opportunities for trainees who are underrepresented in medicine. This article compiles the ongoing DEI initiatives in the American Academy of Derma-tology, Women's Dermatologic Society, Association of Professors of Dermatology Society, Society for Investigative Dermatology, Skin of Color Society, American So-ciety for Dermatologic Surgery, The Dermatology Section of the National Medical Association, and Society for Pediatric Dermatology.

The importance of skin of color and diversity, equity, and inclusion (DEI) started to be recognized in the late 1990s. Since then, because of the advocacy and effort of several highly visible leaders in dermatology, noticeable progress has been achieved. Leadership lessons learned for successful implementation of DEI include the following: (1) commitment by and continued engagement of highly visible leaders; (2) engagement of other societies in dermatology; (3) engagement of derma-tology department leaders and educators; (4) education of the next generation of dermatologists; (5) inclusivity in DEI to include gender and sexual orientation; and (6) cultivation of allies and allyship.

DERMATOLOGIC CLINICS

SERIES OF RELATED INTEREST

Medical Clinics
https://www.medical.theclinics.com/
Immunology and Allergy Clinics
https://www.immunology.theclinics.com/
Clinics in Plastic Surgery
https://www.plasticsurgery.theclinics.com/
Otolaryngologic Clinics
https://www.oto.theclinics.com/

Preface
Diversity, Equity, and Inclusion in Dermatology

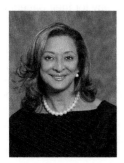

Susan C. Taylor, MD, FAAD
Editor

Of all the forms of inequality, injustice in health care is the most shocking and inhumane.

— *Dr Martin Luther King Jr*

What exactly is diversity, equity, inclusion (DEI), and more importantly, why is it important in medicine and dermatology? The genesis of this *Dermatologic Clinics* is to explore and more deeply understand DEI and its impact on the health and care of our patients, the working and learning environments of dermatologists and trainees, and clinical trial research.

The article in this issue by Mason, "Diversity, Equity, Inclusion and Belonging in Dermatology," provides a foundational understanding of DEI, including definitions and a perspective on the importance of DEI in medicine and dermatology. An argument is made that DEI is essential for excellence in dermatologic care for all patients, serves to address health disparities that exist in marginalized patient populations and provides a healthy and enriched work environment for dermatologists and trainees.

The article by Barbosa delves into "Diversity, Equity, and Inclusion in the Dermatology Workforce and Academic Medicine," and the article by Shinkai et al. focuses on "Diversity and Inclusion in Dermatology Residency," the precursor of the dermatology workforce. The goal of these articles is to understand how and why it is important for the physician workforce to reflect the diversity of the US population and how to begin to achieve this goal. In the article by Barbosa, the subspecialties of pediatric dermatology, dermatopathology and dermatologic surgery are highlighted as even less racially and ethnically diverse than the dermatology workforce as a whole. In the article by Shinkai et al., the authors outline a framework for DEI initiatives at the residency training level, which includes establishing inclusive learning environments and mentoring structures that support residents, as well as instituting improvements in the residency selection process. The authors also discuss the development of curricula to train residents to provide expert care to all patients, and for them to better understand principles of health equity and social determinants of health. This article also initiates a discussion of gender diversity in dermatology and academic medicine.

The article by Murrell and colleagues provides an in-depth look at "Gender Equity in Medicine and Dermatology," highlighting the gains that women have made as academic faculty members and dermatology resident trainees, which is in contrast to the limited number of women in academic leadership positions. The role of gender bias and the dearth of role models are discussed as underlying reasons for these inequities.

An underpinning of the specialty of dermatology is excellence in dermatologic care for all patients. Personal, cultural, and social impediments hinder the attainment of this goal and contribute to health disparities. The articles by Pandya and Rodriguez Jr, Ogunleye, Weir, and Peebles discuss how to begin to overcome some of these impediments. The article by Pandya and Rodriguez Jr reviews

Dermatol Clin 41 (2023) xiii–xv
https://doi.org/10.1016/j.det.2022.12.001

"Cultural Competence and Humility," that practicing dermatologists can incorporate to meet the needs and nuances that occur during racially and ethnically discordant visits between health care providers and patients. The authors emphasize that learning cultural competence and humility are lifelong processes and the fact that it is important to join existing efforts within professional dermatology associations to encourage competence and humility development. They include the idea that improving cultural competence and humility are two ways dermatologists can help lessen the burden of health care disparities.

In the article by Ogunleye, "Unconscious Biases" (also known as implicit biases) are defined as involuntary stereotypes or attitudes held about certain groups of people that may influence behaviors, understandings, and actions, often with unintended detrimental consequences, particularly for diverse populations. Health disparities may partly be attributable to unconscious biases. Implicit bias appears in multiple facets of medical education, training, and promotion with negative effects on diversity and equity efforts. The author discusses evidence (or the lack thereof) supporting the effectiveness of current bias/diversity training programming and the use of standardization and blinding as well as evidence-based methods to reduce implicit bias.

In the clinical setting, both physicians and patients can commit microaggressions or be the targets of microaggression. In "Understanding and Addressing Microaggressions in Medicine" Weir discusses microaggressions, which are aggressions that are delivered unconsciously through words, tone, gestures, or looks, and which convey disparaging sentiments to people of color, women, sexual or gender minority, or other minority groups. Patients who experience microaggression from their provider suffer emotional distress and distrust, resulting in decreased service utilization, reduced treatment compliance, and poorer physical and mental health. Minority group physicians and medical trainees are increasingly the targets of microaggressions committed by patients. This article provides instruction on how to recognize and address microaggressions in the clinical setting and how to create a more supportive and inclusive environment for patients, dermatologists, and our trainees.

A comprehensive discussion of "Achieving Equity for Sexual and Gender Minority Persons in Medicine and Dermatology" occurs in the article by Peebles et al. The authors emphasize the key role that dermatologists play in improving health equity for sexual and gender minority patients through cultivating awareness of how their patients' sexual and gender identity may impact their skin health. They also emphasize that dermatologists must be instrumental in developing sexual and gender minority–inclusive curricula and safe spaces in medical training, promoting workforce diversity, practicing with intersectionality in mind, and engaging in advocacy for their patients, whether it be through daily practice, legislative and/or public policy initiatives, or research.

Structural impediments also hinder the attainment of excellence in dermatologic care for all patients. The articles by Bowers and colleagues provide an understanding of the principles of social determinants of health and health equity as they pertain to dermatology, particularly for marginalized patient populations. Social determinants of health are the nonmedical factors, such as housing, education level, access to food and clean water, neighborhood safety, and economic stability, that must be addressed to improve health outcomes and achieve greater health equity. Social Determinants of Health—Part A aims to shed light on how these determinants impact health and their implications on dermatologic health disparities, whereas Part B offers a framework that dermatologists can employ to help address social determinants of health both at the point of care and in the health care system at large. Social determinants of health are shaped by structural determinants of health, and the article by Vasquez and Pritchett discusses the "History of Race and Ethnicity in America," while the article by Allen and Mickel explores race, racism, and structural racism in medicine. These articles provide a framework for understanding "Racial and Ethnic Health Disparities in Dermatology," which is found in the article by Harvey and colleagues. Health disparities are differences in health or disease incidence, prevalence, severity, or disease burden that are experienced by disadvantaged populations. Health disparities are complex and multifactorial and are often linked to social and economic disadvantage. They originate from dynamic interactions of genetic, biologic, environmental, social, economic, and health system–related factors.

To better understand additional principles of health equity, clinical research trials, an essential component of research for determining the safety and efficacy of treatments for medical diseases, are discussed in the article by Elbuluk and Syder, "Racial Disparities in Research and Clinical Trials." Clinical trials have significantly lagged behind in diverse participation across demographic groups, particularly in regard to race and ethnicity. Within dermatologic randomized clinical trials, studies on conditions such as alopecia areata, atopic dermatitis, and acne have been shown to have a significant majority of white participants. In addition, there are a limited number of trials concerning conditions that disproportionately affect patients with skin of color, and a significant number of dermatology studies fail to report data on minority recruitment and enrollment. These gaps negatively impact health equity, and the authors discuss needed efforts for sustained and meaningful change.

In this issue of *Dermatologic Clinics*, several articles support the case for the role of the dermatologist and our professional dermatology associations in building a diverse, equitable, and inclusive environment for patients and colleagues in clinical care, education, and research. The final articles of the issue discuss opportunities to achieve DEI in dermatology, mechanisms to address health inequities, as well as racial and ethnic intolerance and discrimination. The article by Ferguson and Munjal details the ongoing efforts and DEI initiatives being undertaken by US professional dermatology associations. Each organization had demonstrated a strong commitment to initiatives designed to improve patient care for people of all backgrounds, reduce health disparities, and increase physician education and the number of diverse dermatologists and trainees. Finally, the article by Lim outlines "Steps Leaders Can Take to Increase Diversity, Enhance Inclusion, and Achieve Equity" in dermatology. The author highlights the noticeable progress that has been achieved by the advocacy and effort of several highly visible leaders in dermatology and reviews six key leadership lessons learned for successful implementation of DEI.

Susan C. Taylor, MD, FAAD
Department of Dermatology
Perelman School of Medicine
University of Pennsylvania
3400 Civic Center Boulevard
South Tower, 7-768
Philadelphia, PA 19104, USA

E-mail address:
Susan.Taylor@pennmedicine.upenn.edu

Diversity, Equity, Inclusion and Belonging in Dermatology

Bonnie Simpson Mason, MD[a],*, Candrice Heath, MD[b],
Jennifer Parker, MD, PhD, MPH[b], Kamaria Coleman, BS[c]

KEYWORDS

- Diversity • Equity • Inclusion • Belonging • Healthcare • Dermatology

KEY POINTS

- Improving diversity, equity, inclusion, and belonging (DEIB) in deramtology leads to more accurate diagnoses; improved patient satisfaction, compliance, and outcomes; and overall decreased inequities in health and healthcare.
- To achieve a productive diverse workforce supportive and inclusive clinical and learning environments are required. The absence of emphasis on DEIB negatively impacts patients, practitioners, and the overall practice of dermatology.
- Efforts to address inequities require active implementation of equity practices and includive actions from specialty organizations and institutions that are responsible for education and care delivery.

INTRODUCTION

Diversity, equity, inclusion, and belonging (DEIB) are topics that are gaining much recognition in all specialties of medicine, especially in dermatology. The cause is multifactorial and is evident by a stark increase in DEIB literature, partially stemming from the social unrest in 2020 that occurred after the murder of George Floyd. It is also imperative to note that the stark health disparities *highlighted* in the United States during the height of the COVID-19 pandemic, coupled with the growing organizational interest, has started to recognize that efforts to address DEIB are not only needed—they are necessary. A marked increase in DEIB articles in PubMed supports this. In 2020, there were 193 articles on diversity, equity, and inclusion, and in 2021, this number more than doubled to 483. The literature highlights the both importance and the benefits of DEIB in medicine and health care. Most frequently cited benefits of increasing DEIB include producing more accurate diagnoses and improved patient satisfaction, increased patient compliance, publishing more articles with more citations, improved equipment to address health disparities, and an increase in the production and clinical studies that can benefit patients.[1,2]

Overview of the Relationship Among Diversity, Equity, Inclusion, and Belonging

Increasing diversity of the physician workforce has been a long-standing goal, which aims to have the composition of those rendering care be reflective of the composition of those cared for. This goal of parity of representation spans across categories of race and ethnicities, language preferences, abilities, geography, just to name a few indices of diversity. The long-term goal of establishing a diverse workforce is to be able to render better, culturally specific care resulting in better

[a] American College of Surgeons, 20 F Street, Northwest, Suite 1000, Washington, DC 20001, USA;
[b] Departmenf of Dermatology, Temple University Lewis Katz School of Medicine, 3401 N. Broad Sreet, Suite B500, Philadelphia, PA 19140, USA; [c] Southern Illinois University School of Medicine, 801 N. Rutledge Street, Springfield, IL 62702, USA
* Corresponding author.
E-mail address: DrBonnieMason@gmail.com

Dermatol Clin 41 (2023) 239–248
https://doi.org/10.1016/j.det.2022.08.002

outcomes and decreased inequities in health and health care for patients.

However, focusing solely on increasing representation of diverse groups in medicine without creating supportive, inclusive clinical and learning environments, through the implementation of equity practices can be detrimental to members of the workforce and ultimately to patients. Equity, as described by Dr Camara Jones,[3] looks to optimize the workplace, for example, clinical and learning environments, for those in the workforce, for example, students, trainees, practicing physicians, staff and leaders. According to Dr Jones, in order to achieve this equity goal, the following are required:

- All persons and populations are valued equally,
- Historical and current injustices must be recognized and rectified, and
- Resources should be provided according to need.

Implementing practices that satisfy these aspects of equity learning and clinical environments serves to create an inclusive culture that actively honors and supports differing voices, talents, and experiences as being necessary contributors to excellence in the environment. The result for all individuals and groups within the workforce is a sense of belonging that allows all members of the workforce to present themselves authentically and subsequently perform maximally. Maximal performance in health care ultimately benefits the patient now that both quality of care and environmental safety are the positive downstream effects of ongoing development and implementation of meaningful and sustainable equity practices.

Wanting to belong is a basic human desire and some would argue that it is a necessity. It describes a feeling of being connected socially in a positive way to a group of others.[4–6] DEIB critically affect patients, physicians, clinicians, and the overall practice of medicine. Racism, microaggressions, and unconscious bias prevent some from feeling like they belong. This yearning to belong is a psychological need that improves well-being.[7] A positive well-being is necessary to serve our patients, who if marginalized, are also influenced negatively by the absence of emphasis on DEIB. We are all negatively influenced by social determinants of health and disparities, whether personally or indirectly.

Thus, DEIB efforts can be categorized into 3 main areas of impact: patients, practitioners, and the overall practice of dermatology (**Fig. 1**). These efforts to diversify the physician workforce in every specialty must be coupled with equity practices that yield inclusive health care and learning environments that lead to a culture of belonging, thereby optimizing access, patient safety, and quality of care rendered.

As these concepts are not mutually exclusive, efforts to address inequities in health and health care that have not considered this integrated approach have unsurprisingly fallen short as evidenced by persisting and disparate morbidity and mortality of diverse US populations.

Background

Inequities in access and delivery of care due to structural and systemic racism and the resulting social and legal determinants of health continue to result in disparities in health and health care primarily for historically and currently marginalized populations in the United States. In 2002, Unequal Treatment published by the Institute of Medicine cited that in every chronic disease category, Black Americans suffered disproportionately greater than White Americans. Specifically, racial and ethnic differences in health care, not otherwise attributable to known factors such as access to care, were consistently found across a wide range of disease areas and clinical services. Even when clinical factors, such as stage of disease presentation, comorbidities, age, and severity of disease are considered, disparities between black and White patients persisted irrespective of the clinical settings in which care was rendered, including public and private hospitals, teaching and nonteaching hospitals, and so forth.[8] Ultimately, the literature shows that disparities in care are associated with higher mortality among minorities.[9,10]

Studies demonstrate that people of color do not have optimal access to medical screenings, interventions, and are at risk for surgical

The 3 P's

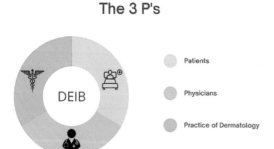

Patients

Physicians

Practice of Dermatology

Fig. 1. Patients, Physicians, and the Practice of Dermatology (Medicine) can represent 3 categories of impact for efforts in diversity, equity, inclusion, and belonging.

complications.[11] Black patients are 30% less likely to receive revascularization during coronary angioplasty and 40% less likely to receive coronary bypass surgery. Black women are 40% more likely to die from breast cancer than their White counterparts. Black and Hispanic youth are more likely to die from diabetes complications.[1] In fact, the adverse effect on patients remains no matter where they are engaging with our current medical system. Lack of health equity is prevalent in access to medical screenings, rates of surgical complications, and even treatment in the hospital.[1,11]

There are also several examples within dermatology highlighting the disparities in health outcomes among patients of color. In one study by Barbieri and colleagues, almost 30,000 patients were examined for associations between patient demographic and socioeconomic characteristics with the health care utilization and acne treatment during 1 year of follow-up.[12] The findings revealed that although non-Hispanic Black patients were more likely to be seen by a dermatologist (odds ratio 1.20, 95% CI 1.09–1.31) than non-Hispanic White patients, they received fewer prescriptions for acne medications (Incidence Rate Ratio 0.89, 95% CI 0.84–0.95).[12] In addition, Black patients were more likely to receive topical retinoids and topical antibiotics compared with oral antibiotics, spironolactone, and isotretinoin.[12] Similar disparities are seen with management of psoriasis in Black patients. Retrospective review of diagnosis confirmed psoriasis patients at 4 institutions revealed that psoriatic skin disease was more severe in Black patients compared with White patients (Psoriasis Area and Severity Index 8.4 vs 5.5) with greater psychological impact and impaired quality of life. However, use of biological therapies was greater in White patients than Black patients (42.2% vs 13.3%).[13] A similar phenomenon is noted in the pediatric dermatology population.[14]

A systematic review of racial, ethnic, and socioeconomic health disparities showed increased risk of impaired access to dermatologic care, more severe atopic dermatitis, ineffective sun protection education, and advanced stage of skin cancer at diagnosis.[14] As an example, the review showed Black and Hispanic children are less likely to see providers, have more severe disease, more persistent disease, greater school absenteeism, and more likely to need multiple visits for good disease control.[14] Medicaid insurance increases the likelihood of emergency department usage and reduces access to dermatologists, who often do not accept Medicaid insurance. There are more comorbidities in non-White patients.[14] There are also ongoing racial disparities in melanoma. Qian

and colleagues analyzed 381,035 patients from the SEER registry.

Racial disparity worsened from before the year 2000 to 2010 or later for Hispanic ($P < .001$), non-Hispanic Blacks ($P = .024$), and non-Hispanic Asian Pacific Islanders ($P < .001$) patients.[15] Across all minority groups, patients with localized disease suffered increasing disparity. Of those with regional and distant disease, Hispanic patients experienced worsening disparity.[15]

In addition, the effects of structural and systemic racism are evident in medical education at all levels, as well. In 2016, researchers at the University of Virginia investigated the beliefs and knowledge of their students and residents based on race.[16] In this study, 222 White medical students from the University of Virginia were asked to read made-up cases; one about a black patient and the other about a White patient and then rate their perceived pain on a scale from 1 to 10. These students were then asked to evaluate 15 "facts" regarding biological differences between the races. All but 4 of the facts were fake. The actual facts were that black patients were more at risk for heart disease and stroke, had higher bone densities than Whites, and were less at risk for spinal cord diseases. The researchers made up facts, which included Blacks' nerve endings are less sensitive than Whites' and Blacks' skin is thicker than Whites'. Fifty percent of the students thought that at least 1 of the fake statements was "possibly, probably, or definitely true." Those who believed the fake facts were more likely to show a "racial bias" in how they assessed *and* treated the pain of the White and Black patients. A hundred and six non-White students had no correlation. Moreover, the initial results showed that 40% of participants held thoughts that black patients' skin was thicker than that of White patients. After an educational intervention that addressed these same points was implemented, 25% of participants continued to answer these questions incorrectly. The clinical implications resulting from lack of knowledge or right held thoughts belie studies, which reveal that Blacks and Latino receive:

- Less pain medication,
- Fewer and later referrals for specialty oncologic care, and
- Fewer elective operative procedures.

The medical student-based study results of perceived differences black and white skin, uniquely, applies dermatology. The basis for the study of skin disease is visual and has been historically described and depicted on white skin, thus

Table 1
Patients

Culture of Belonging Scenario	Culture of Belonging Response Option 1	Response Option 2
A patient of different skin tone, race, ethnicity, or hair texture from the physician enters the room. Patient stares skeptically at the physician during the introduction	After introducing themselves, the physician states, "I know that there is a perception that because I am [insert race here] I am not equipped to handle your concerns. I can assure you that I have been trained on your skin type. I look forward to working together. How do you feel about that?" Patient thanks the physician for opening the visit with that acknowledgment. The patient leaves the visit satisfied, feeling valued, and listened to with a deeper knowledge of their skin condition and with appreciation for their dermatologist. They look forward to following up with this same provider	Approaching visits with cultural humility is the foundation for patient belonging. Although obtaining information for the history of present illness, the questions asked demonstrate the physician's insights into the patient's personal experience with darker skin tones or naturally tightly coiled hair. In absence of this knowledge, as a premise of cultural humility, physician creates atmosphere of unintentional harm. Offering options for treatments—variety of vehicles and frequencies that fit with patient preferences[22]

Culture of Belonging Scenario	Not Culture of Belonging Response Option 1	Response Option 2
Patient of different skin tone, race, ethnicity, or hair texture from the physician enters the room. Patient stares skeptically at the physician during the introduction	After introducing themselves, the physician notices the patient skeptically looking at them. The physician proceeds with the examination, offers a diagnosis, and ends the visit. Patient asks the provider if they are sure of the diagnosis based on their race and skin complexion. Provider responds that they have had the proper training and race does not influence the current diagnosis The patient leaves the visit unsatisfied, feeling disregarded and unlistened to, with no understanding of their skin condition. They decide to change providers	In a study by Gorbatenko-Roth, patients reported a dermatologist *who does not engage in the physical examination*[20] When examining of the hair of a patient with tightly coiled hair, approaching with cultural humility is advised.[22] Additionally, patient–dermatologist racial concordance was preferred but not necessary for a positive patient experience[20] Creating a culture of belonging would allow dermatologists of all races and ethnicities to acknowledge that there are perceived biases around race, which is a social construct. However, these biases are not concrete and can be changed

Table description: As you can see in the scenarios above, a culture of belonging focuses on creating an environment where practitioners and patients have the ability to freely discuss these issues and create a solution together to move forward. The principals from the above scenario can be applied to racially discordant patients and overall interactions with all patients. Ultimately, the ultimate goal of the interaction would be to advance and strengthen the patient–physician relationship.

perpetuating health inequities before a diagnosis is even made. This limited provision of diverse representation of the appearance of pathologic condition on black and brown skin serves to disadvantage skin specialists and ultimately negatively affects the subsequent care delivered to delay or failure to diagnose disease. In dermatology, there is a significant and well-documented lack of training in skin of color in both textbooks and online resources. This disparity in medical education adversely affects dermatologist practitioners and patients. If dermatology is now only increasing the skin of color learning opportunities, we can only predict that other specialties lag behind, as well. With 7% of all primary care visits having a dermatologic focus,[17] physicians and practitioners who are exposed to fewer skin of color examples results in less opportunity to develop the crucial skill of pattern recognition. Patients are adversely affected because the provider may not have had exposure to the specific condition seen in the patient's skin tone. This could result in delayed, missed, and even misdiagnosis.[18] Combined with the difficulty marginalized communities face accessing dermatologists, patients of color are greatly impacted by the paucity of skin of color specific training across specialties.[19]

Research shows that Black patients seen by a dermatologist trained in skin of color report increased satisfaction compared with prior experiences. The improvement in satisfaction is linked to

Table 2
Physicians

Culture of Belonging Scenario	Culture of Belonging Response Option 1	Response Option 2
A resident is experiencing symptoms of burnout. They have fallen behind on their notes, have not been appropriately answering consults, and have been arriving to work late	The program director is aware of the incidents with the resident. They set up a meeting with them to discuss efficiency, dealing with life stressors, and offer to pair them with a senior resident for a few shifts to observe their workflow. After a few weeks of working with the senior resident and weekly meetings with the program director, the resident has been more efficient at work, offering timely consults, and arriving to work on time	According to Youmans et al,[23] building an inclusive environment that focuses on belonging for all can help increase recruitment and retention, decrease isolation, and lack of belonging for underrepresented in medicine trainees[23]
Culture of Belonging Scenario	**Not Culture of Belonging Response Option 1**	**Response Option 2**
A resident is experiencing symptoms of burnout. They have fallen behind on their notes, have not been appropriately answering consults, and have been arriving to work late	The fellow residents of the resident who is falling behind, talk behind their back about their slack and need to "pick up the pace." They discuss the resident issues with the program director who keeps the complaints in a file. At the end of the year, the resident is told that they need a year of remediation if they wish to continue with the program	According to Shanefelt, dermatology has the highest increase in the prevalence of burnout, increasing from 37% in 2011 to 57% in 2014.[24] Burnout is not limited to practicing physicians but affects trainees as well. The 2 most contributing factors to burnout were autonomy and appropriate work–life balance[25]

Table description: Creating an environment that focuses on belonging would provide ways for burnout in physicians, trainees, and students to be identified and then mitigated appropriately. Possible solutions are not widely applicable to all solutions but require an intense focus on individual needs.

several factors including practitioner knowledge about black skin and hair and a culturally sensitive interaction style. It is imperative to mention that patient–dermatologist racial concordance was preferred but not necessary for a positive patient experience.[20] Creating a culture of belonging would allow dermatologists of all races and ethnicities to acknowledge that there are perceived biases around race, which is a social construct.

However, these biases are not concrete and can be changed. A physician workforce with such beliefs will only continue to deliver inequitable care unless the foundation of medical education actively works to address medical educational curricula in all specialties.

In dermatology, a lack of diversity, equity, and inclusion is present at several levels including

Table 3
Practice of dermatology

Culture of Belonging Scenario	Culture of Belonging Response Option 1	Response Option 2
A survey is conducted that asks medical trainees to identify melanoma on darker skin. More than 50% of participants miss the diagnosis of melanoma on non–White/darker skin	After getting the results of the survey, the program director of the residency adds images on skin of color for commonly missed diagnosis in darker skin. Images are also added for the most common dermatology images on darker skin. By the end of the residency, training residents feel adequately prepared to both diagnose and treat diseases on skin of color individuals	The misdiagnosis of melanoma should not be the only focus on education. In fact, this diagnosis can be used to discuss health disparities in dermatology. According to Youmans, creating safe and open spaces for dialog is essential for building inclusive environments.[23] By creating open dialog, leaders can provide spaces for trainees to reflect on formative parts of their identity. In this way, trainees from all backgrounds can grow in safe spaces in an open and inclusive environment[23]

Culture of Belonging Scenario	Not Culture of Belonging Response Option 1	Response Option 2
A survey is conducted that asks medical trainees to identify melanoma on darker skin. More than 50% of participants miss the diagnosis of melanoma on non–White/darker skin	After getting the results of the survey, the program director of the residency decides that the survey was not an adequate representation of the training that residents received. They decide not to create any specific educational objectives and thought that the patient population is diverse enough to provide the needed number for sufficient pattern recognition. At the end of residency, the trainees feel indifferent in their ability to diagnose and treat diseases on skin of color individuals	According to Buster, although melanoma is more common in non-Hispanic Whites and individuals with high SES, Blacks and those with low SES present with more clinically advanced disease or suffer from increased mortality. In order to create a culture of belonging in dermatology, there must be advances in screening and detection that allow those with a lesser incidence of melanoma to be adequately detected[19]

Table description: Creating an inclusive environment that emphasizes belonging for all requires intentionality. In order to foster the space for belonging our current systems must be open to creating systems that provide space for all to be seen and resources for all members to be adequately accessed.

Levels of Accountability

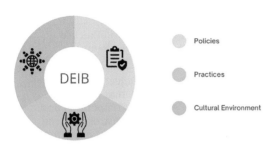

Policies

Practices

Cultural Environment

Fig. 2. Those in leadership roles at specialty, institutional, and departmental levels have the opportunity to implement and be accountable for affecting structural and systemic changes in DEIB at the policy, practice, and ultimately the cultural environment (clinical and learning) levels.

recruitment, residency retention, faculty development, dermatology workforce, and beyond.[21]

Addressing Inequities

Efforts to address inequities require the active implementation of equity practices and inclusive actions from specialty organizations and institutions responsible for education and care delivery, which starts with individual commitments from leaders, faculty, staff, trainees, and students. These efforts are only capable in driving transformational change if coupled with institutional/organizational, as well as individual accountability.

The goal of creating a medical environment that recognizes diversity, equity, and inclusion is to create a culture of belonging for both patients and practitioners. By creating a culture of belonging, we will then be able to improve our practice of medicine.

DEI efforts abound, belonging is, however, the missing piece. For learners and practicing physicians in medicine, the sense of belonging could be replaced by feelings of isolation. We fear that, with increased DEI efforts, doing the work to succeed will result only in a shift in numbers but leave that majority still feeling isolated. Dermatology is among the least diverse specialties.

Only a minority of the members of the dermatology workforce identify as racial and ethnic minorities, and/or sexual and gender minorities.

Table 4
Recommendations for accountability measures for leadership at all levels

Levels of Accountability for DEI and Belonging	Specialty	Hospital Systems/ Institution	Physicians in Training and in Practice— (Academic and Nonhospital Based)
Policies	Beyond written statements alone, leadership commitment from specialty associations and board certifying bodies should be reflected in strategic planning and resource allocation in budgeting Hold board of directors members accountable for operationalizing DEIB efforts at all levels	Ensure that system and institutional DEI commitments are verbalized and represented throughout one's campus Confidential feedback mechanisms for patients and health-care workforce should be implemented	Listen, inquire, and advocate for policies promoting equity practices, eg, parity in representation and pay equity
Practices	Implement standardized demographic data collections to determine recruitment, retention/attrition	Bias response strategies should be planned, rehearsed, and socialized enterprise-wide	Commit to engaging all individuals, especially those from diverse backgrounds

(continued on next page)

Table 4 (*continued*)			
Levels of Accountability for DEI and Belonging	Specialty	Hospital Systems/ Institution	Physicians in Training and in Practice— (Academic and Nonhospital Based)
Culture/Environment	Perform environmental/ culture assessments at the undergraduate medical education, graduate medical education, and continuing medical education levels to measure impact of DEI efforts	Espouse core values prioritizing the creation safe, equitable, and inclusive learning and clinical environments for workforce and patients	Reject cultural norms that promote competition and mistrust. Instead invest in cultural humility, and collegial accountability with support

Diversity, equity, inclusion, and belonging are important topics that affect patients, providers, and the overall practice of medicine. By creating an inclusive culture that is reflective of DEI, we aim to cultivate an environment that can help improve patient outcomes, access to health care, decrease burnout in providers, and provide a space for everyone to feel valued, seen, and ultimately provide a space for everyone to belong.

The task of DEI and fostering belonging must be comprehensive. From approaching patients and colleagues with cultural humility to harnessing the power of dermatology organizations, this has to be a united leadership priority. By creating an inclusive culture that is truly reflective of DEIB, physicians and the health-care workforce must become educated and be trained on with the requisite skills to the aim is to cultivate an environment that helps to improve patient outcomes, access to health care, decrease burnout among health-care team members, and provide a space for everyone to feel valued, seen, and ultimately provide a space for everyone to belong.

Case-Scenarios in Addressing Inequities

The following case scenarios are examples of lived experiences that are evident in patients (**Table 1**), physicians (**Table 2**), and the practice of dermatology (**Table 3**). Along with each scenario are suggested approaches to address the described inequalities.

SUMMARY

Addressing continued inequities in medicine, and especially in dermatology, requires a strategic approach and meaningful actions that will yield and result in sustainable change in our medical, clinical, and learning environments. This will require a paradigm shift likened to the reverse ideation approach, which will require that leadership at the specialty, institutional, and physician levels be held responsible and accountable for the culture shift necessary to create safe equitable and inclusive environments for the health-care workforce such that better quality of care can be rendered to all patients. Heretofore, most solutions-based actions and programs in DEI have focused on developing and edifying the diverse learner or faculty member. Alternatively, accountability rests with the entities that wield the power and ability and authority to shift culture change such that the diverse learner, faculty member, and patient can receive equitable access to care and educational resources in environments within a culture of belonging. The onus and accountability must rest on the shoulders of the entities that have both the willingness and authority to allocate resources, set strategic direction and institute attainable metrics that leadership at the levels of the board of directors of specialty associations, hospital systems, and academic institutions must be held liable for through frequent and transparent communication of impact and outcomes (**Fig. 2**).

The following are recommendations for accountability measures for leadership at all levels for those seeking to achieve a culture of belonging in all aspects of medicine (**Table 4**).

CLINICS CARE POINTS

- Review of diversity evidenced-based research specific to healthcare revealed positive associations between diversity, care quality, and financial performance.

- Surveys of minority dermatology patients reveal patients prefer race concordant dermatologists alluding to the necessity of diversifying the dermatology workforce and strengthening of cultural competency in training to offset the adverse effects.

- Dermatologic disparities which need to be addressed have been identified in studies examining outcomes in patients of color with acne, psoriasis, atopic dermatitis, and melanoma.

- To establish a fruitful diverse workforce a sense of belonging is required. Social belonging exerpiments data have demonstrated increased well-being, improved academic performance, and health outcomes for the participants..

DISCLOSURE

The authors have nothing to disclose.

REFERENCES

1. Gomez LE, Bernet P. Diversity improves performance and outcomes. J Natl Med Assoc 2019; 111:383–92.
2. Swartz TH, Palermo AGS, Masur SK, et al. The science and value of diversity: closing the gaps of our understanding of inclusion and diversity. J Infect Dis 2019;220:S33–41.
3. Jones CP. Systems of power, axes of inequity: parallel, intersections, braiding the strands. Med Care 2014;52:S71–5.
4. Baumeister RF, Brewer LE, Tice DM, et al. Thwarting the need to belong: understanding the interpersonal and inner effects of social exclusion. Soc Personal Psychol Compass 2007;1:506–20.
5. Salles A, Wright RC, Milam L, et al. Social belonging as a predictor of surgical well- being and attrition. J Surg Educ 2019;76:370–7.
6. Walton GM Cohen GL. A brief social-belonging intervention improves academic and health outcomes of minority students. Science 2011;331:1147–51.
7. Greenway KH, Cruwys T, Hallam SA, et al. Social identities promote well- being because they satisfy global psychological needs. Eur J Soc Psychol 2015;46:294–307.
8. Smedley BD, Stith AV, Nelson AR. Unequal treatment: confronting racial and ethnic disparities in health care. Washington, DC: National Academy Press (US); 2003.
9. Bach PB, Cramer LD, Warren JL, et al. Racial differences in the treatment of early-stage lung cancer. N Engl J Med 1999;341:1198–205.
10. Peterson ED, Shaw LK, DeLong ER, et al. Racial variation in the use of coronary-revascularization procedures—are the differences real? Do they matter? N Engl J Med 1997;336:480–6.
11. McBean AM, Gornick M. Differences by race in the rates of procedures performed in hospitals for Medicare beneficiaries. Health Care Financ Rev 1994;15: 77–90.
12. Barbieri JS, Shin DB, Wang S, et al. Association of race/ethnicity and sex with differences in health care use and treatment for acne. JAMA Dermatol 2020;156:312–9.
13. Kerr GS, Qaiyumi S, Richards J, et al. Psoriasis and psoriatic arthritis in African-American patients the need to measure disease burden. Clin Rheumatol 2015;34:1753–9.
14. Kuo A, Silverberg N, Faith EF, et al. A systematic scoping review of racial, ethnic, socioeconomic health disparities in pediatric dermatology. Pediatr Dermatol 2021;38:6–12.
15. Qian Y, Johannet P, Sawyers A, et al. The ongoing racial disparities in melanoma: an analysis of the surveillance, epidemiology, and end results database (1975-2016). J Am Acad Dermatol 2021;84: 1585–93.
16. Hoffman KM, Trawalter S, Axt JR, et al. Racial bias in pain assessment, treatment recommendations, and false beliefs about biological differences in Blacks and Whites. PNAS 2016;113:4296–301.
17. Ramsay DL, Fox AB. The ability of primary care physicians to recognize common dermatoses. Arch Dermatol 1981;117:620–2.
18. Slaught C, Mary P, Chang AY, et al. Novel education modules addressing the underrepresentation of skin of color in dermatology training. J Cutan Med Surg 2022;26:17–24.
19. Buster KJ, Stevens EI, Elmer's CA. Dermatologic health disparities. Dermatol Clin 2012;30:53-vii.
20. Gorbatenko- Roth K, Prose N, Kundu RV, et al. Assessment of Black patients' perception of their dermatology care. JAMA Dermatol 2019;155:1129–34.
21. Akhiyat S, Cardwell L, Sokumbi O. Why dermatology is the second least diverse specialty in medicine: How did we get here? Clin Dermatol 2020;38:310–5.
22. Grayson C, Heath C. An approach to examining tightly coiled hair among patients with hair loss in race-discordant patient-physician interactions. JAMA Dermatol 2021;157:505–6.

23. Youmans QR, Maldanado M, Essien UR, et al. Building inclusion and belonging in training environments. J Grad Med Educ 2022;14:333–4.

24. Shanafelt TD, Hasan O, Dyrbye LN, et al. Changes in burnout and satisfaction with work-life balance in physicians and the general US working population between 2011 and 2014. Mayo Clin Proc 2015;90:1600–13.

25. Marchalik R, Marchalik D, Wang H, et al. Drivers and sequelae of burnout in U.S. dermatology trainees. Int J Womens Dermatol 2021;7:780–6.

Diversity in the Dermatology Workforce and in Academic Medicine

Karina Grullon, BS[a,1], Victoria Barbosa, MD, MPH, MBA[b,*]

KEYWORDS

- Diversity - Health disparities - Physician workforce - Academic dermatology

KEY POINTS

- Having a physician workforce that reflects the US population is an important step toward addressing health disparities.
- The dermatology workforce is not representative of the increasingly diverse US population.
- Dermatology subspecialties are less diverse than the dermatology workforce as a whole.
- Gender diversity has improved in academic dermatology, whereas racial and ethnic diversity has not.

INTRODUCTION

Health disparities are preventable differences in health, disease burden, or health care that stem from broader social, economic, and/or systemic inequities. It is well established that health disparities exist for members of marginalized communities, including people belonging to racial or ethnic minority groups and people who are gender or sexual minorities.[1] Examples can be found in many specialties of medicine. For instance, there continue to be higher rates of both maternal and infant mortality among black women and children compared with whites.[2,3] And although Hispanics have a lower death rate compared with whites overall, they are 50% more likely to die from diabetes and have a higher rate of liver disease.[4] Health care disparities exist within dermatology as well. Blacks and Hispanics have higher likelihood of having atopic dermatitis persisting into adulthood and tend to have more severe hidradenitis suppurativa. These groups also have diagnostic delay, longer times to definitive treatment,

and poorer outcomes than white patients for melanoma.[5] In addition to these preventable inequities, care for patients with skin of color (SOC) requires the ability to recognize dermatologic diseases in different skin types, experience managing conditions seen disproportionately in patients with SOC, and cultural sensitivity and humility.

Although improving care for patients with SOC and reducing health disparities will require a multipronged approach, having a diverse physician workforce that reflects the composition of the US population is critical to improving the care of all patients for several reasons. Physicians from groups underrepresented in medicine (URiM) are more likely to treat patients of color and serve underserved communities. Patients from URiM groups report preference for race-concordant dyads with their physician and report higher levels of trust and higher satisfaction when they are in race-concordant dyads. Also, a diverse workforce expands the cultural competency of physicians treating patients.[6,7]

Diversity within academic medicine is particularly important. Academic dermatologists are

The authors have no conflicts of interest relevant to this article. Dr V. Barbosa serves as consultant and advisory board member for Eli Lilly and has served on advisory boards for Vichy Laboratories and UCB Pharmaceuticals in the last year.

[a] University of Chicago Pritzker School of Medicine; [b] University of Chicago Medicine Section of Dermatology, 5841 South Maryland Avenue, MC5067, L518B, Chicago, IL 60637, USA

[1] Present address: 121 West Central Avenue, Maywood, NJ 07607.

* Corresponding author.

E-mail address: vbarbosa@uchicago.edu

Dermatol Clin 41 (2023) 249–256
https://doi.org/10.1016/j.det.2022.10.005

both educators and role models for medical students, residents, and fellows. As such they are tasked with preparing the next generation of physicians to enter the dermatology workforce ready to deliver quality care that is compassionate, patient-centered, and appropriately attentive to the needs of an increasingly diverse patient population. Improving diversity within academic dermatology can help the specialty achieve excellence in medical education and deliver the highest quality care for all.[8] Multiple studies have shown that increasing diversity in academic medicine helps to reduce health care disparities and improves patient outcomes while enhancing the patient experience and improving population health.[9,10]

Composition of the Dermatology Workforce

From the late 1970s through the early 2000s, the literature on the dermatology workforce focused mainly on physician shortage and on concerns about the geographic distribution of dermatologists. The workforce discourse shifted in 2016 when Pandya and colleagues[11] published the seminal study that demonstrated that dermatology was the second least diverse specialty in the House of Medicine. At that time, blacks made up 12.8% of the US population but only 3% of US dermatologists. Hispanics made up 16.3% of the US population but only 4.2% of US dermatologists. In addition, the discrepancy between the US population and the composition of dermatologists was widening.[11] One can expect that even with the significant attention being drawn to the disparities highlighted in this study, change will be slow given the relatively small number of dermatology residency graduates each year. In 2020 there were just 538 first year dermatology residency positions offered.[12] So even with increasing percentages of URiM residents becoming dermatologists, it will take years for those increases to impact the racial and ethnic distribution of the more than 12,000 practicing dermatologists closer to parity with the composition of the United States.[13]

Little is known about the specific characteristics, challenges, or needs of URiM dermatologists as a group or compared with non-URiM dermatologists. In a survey of 100 dermatologists and trainees, URiM dermatologists were more likely to be born outside the United States; these dermatologists were also 6.5 times more likely to have attended a private medical institution and 4.2 times more likely to have received need-based financial aid compared with their non-URiM counterparts. There was a significant association between being a URiM dermatologist and having had a mentor who was also a URiM dermatologist. Black physicians in

particular were significantly more likely to pursue a master's degree before or during medical school than nonblack physicians. Also, black dermatologists were more likely to have identified interest in dermatology as a career before medical school compared with nonblack physicians. These data provide an important starting point for insights into the URiM dermatologist population.[14]

Workforce data pertaining to sexual and gender minority (SGM) dermatologists is similarly sparse. Most of the limited SGM literature focuses on the dermatologic needs of SGM patients and on resident education rather than on the characteristics or needs of practicing physicians. Mori and colleagues[15] conducted a survey examining the self-identified race, sexual orientation, and specialty choice of graduating medical students from 2016 to 2019. Of the 58,572 respondents who provided data on sexual orientation and intended specialty, 6.3% identified as SGM. Of the 1373 respondents who specifically noted dermatology as their intended specialty, 5.9% identified as SMG. Interestingly, whereas 12.1% of men who were dermatology bound identified as SGM, only 1.9% of women medical school graduates who were dermatology bound identified as SGM. Dermatology had the lowest percentage of SGM women entering the field of any medical specialty.[15]

Women now make up 51% of practicing dermatologists and have reached parity with the US population.[13] However, there are important differences between practicing men and women. A survey of 421 dermatologists revealed that although there was no difference in practice types between women and men, a higher percentage of men worked more than 40 hours per week and men saw on average 22 more patients per week than their female counterparts. Among men and women who worked more than 40 hours per week, women earned less than men.[16] There were also gender differences in practice locations noted. Women were more likely to practice in areas with a higher proportion of Democratic voters and less likely to practice in rural areas.[17] The issue of gender diversity must be further considered in the dermatologic subspecialties and among academic faculty where disparities become more apparent. The characteristics of the dermatology workforce discussed thus far are summarized in **Box 1**.

Diversity in the Dermatology Subspecialties

The lack of diversity in dermatology is particularly evident in the subspecialties of pediatric dermatology, dermatopathology, and dermatologic surgery. In all 3 fields, published research focuses on racial and ethnic diversity and on women,

Box 1
Summary of dermatology workforce characteristics

12,505 practicing dermatologists

51% Women

3% Black

4.2% Hispanic

Second least racially/ethnically diverse specialty in medicine

12.1% of men entering dermatology identify as SGM

1.9% of women entering dermatology identify as SGM

Lowest percentage of SGM women entering of any specialty

with no published data on SGM physicians. And, as with general dermatology workforce data, research is limited.

Although women are well represented in pediatric dermatology, people from URiM groups are not. In a survey of the 336 actively practicing board-certified pediatric dermatologists, 78.6% were women.[18] A recent study published by the Pediatric Dermatology Research Alliance (PeDRA) evaluated self-reported data from its 464 active and trainee members. Similar to the data from the study of actively practicing pediatric dermatologists, 77% were women. Of the 283 who reported data on race and ethnicity, 64.7% were white, 20.1% were Asian/Pacific Islander, 9.5% were Hispanic/Latino, 5.3% were black/African American, and 0.4% were Native American/Alaskan Native. This study illustrated disparities not only in the URiM pediatric dermatology workforce but also in grant funding and society leadership. Of the 51 people who received grants from PeDRA between 2016 and 2021, 35 also reported race. Of those who reported, 71.4% of grant recipients were white, 20% were Asian/Pacific Islander, 5.7% were Hispanic/Latino, and 2.9% identified as Native American/Alaskan Native. None were black. Looking at the society's committee members, 68% of positions were held by whites, 27% by Asian/Pacific Islanders, and 5% by Hispanic/Latinos. There were no black committee members. The board of directors was 80% white and 20% Asian/Pacific Islander. There were no black, Hispanic/Latino, or Native American/Alaskan Native people on the board of directors.[19] This observation highlights the fact that just increasing the numbers of URiM dermatologists is not enough; the pediatric dermatology subspecialty

and the specialty of dermatology in general must identify ways to be more inclusive in research, grant funding, and organizational leadership.

In contrast to pediatric dermatology where there is gender diversity but not racial diversity in the workforce, dermatopathology lacks both gender and racial diversity. Suwatee and colleagues[20] conducted a benchmark survey of Fellows of the American Society of Dermatopathology in 2011. Of the 913 fellows 437 completed the survey, for a response rate of 48%; 72.2% of the respondents were men, 84.9% were white, 10.2% were Asian/Pacific Islander, 2.3% Hispanic/Latino, and 0.7% were black. Forty-nine percent had completed a dermatology residency and 24% were working in academics. The academic dermatopathologists were more likely to be female than those in private practice. No follow-up or more recent data have been published.[20]

Dermatologic surgery also lacks gender and racial diversity according to a study that reviewed the demographics of physicians who coded for Mohs micrographic surgery in a review of 2014 Medicare Provider Utilization and Payment Data. This study identified 2240 Mohs surgeons, 48% of whom were members of the American College of Mohs Surgeons (ACMS). It was found that 28.1% of all surgeons were women, with 32.9% of the ACMS member surgeons being women. Of all surgeons, 80.2% were white, 15.3% were Asian/Pacific Islander, 2.6% were Hispanic/Latino, 1.8% were black/African American, and 0.1% were Native American/Alaskan Native. Results were similar when the investigators looked specifically at ACMS member surgeons. In that group, 78.4% were white, 17.3% were Asian/Pacific Islander, 2.1% were Hispanic/Latino, 2.1% were black/African American, and 0.1% were Native American/Alaskan Native.[21]

Fig. 1 compares the racial and ethnic composition of these 3 dermatology subspecialties based on the data from the 3 separate studies just reviewed. It is evident that for all 3 subspecialties, the percentage of URiM physicians falls below parity with the US population.

Workforce data are vital to any specialty. Dermatologists must know where the field stands to be proactive in charting a path forward. Ideally the workforce should be well positioned to meet the needs of all patients. The specialty and subspecialties should be inclusive of women, URiM physicians, and physicians who identify as SGM. One obvious step is to be more inclusive in the process of training new dermatologists; this necessitates having an understanding of the workforce issues specific to academic medicine.

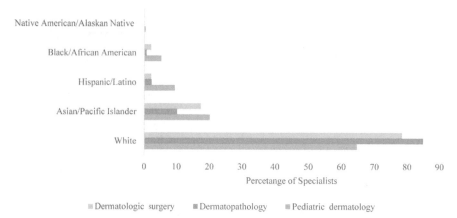

Fig. 1. Dermatology subspecialists by race/ethnicity.

Academic Dermatology Workforce and Specific Challenges

Having a faculty with a wide range of dermatologic expertise and lived experiences not only enhances patient care but also enriches medical student and resident education; this has a ripple effect because these trainees are then better prepared to manage a diverse patient population. Understanding and addressing issues pertaining to faculty diversity are particularly important for this reason. The hierarchy conferred by the faculty appointment level and the often challenging path to promotion are hallmarks of academic medicine and amplify the workforce diversity challenge in academic dermatology.

Faculty data from the AAMC provides a recent snapshot of dermatology faculty composition. In 2021, there were 1606 dermatology faculty members. As illustrated in **Fig. 2**, the vast majority of faculty members are white (66.7%) or Asian (21.1%) with each other group making up only between 0 and 2.9% of the faculty. This data set also provides insight into the rank of the faculty members by race/ethnicity. **Fig. 3** illustrates the faculty rank of the URiM faculty members by race and gender. Numbers for all URiM groups are remarkably small. For Hispanic men, more faculty are at the professor level than any other rank. For black men and women and Hispanic women, the associate level was the most common rank.[22]

Recent studies reveal concerning trends in academic dermatology faculty composition over time. Xierali and colleagues[23] examined the changes in dermatology faculty by race and gender from 1970 to 2018. During that time, the number of dermatology faculty increased from 167 to 1464. Women made significant strides as the number of faculty members grew. The percentage of women faculty increased from 10.8% in 1970 to 51.2% in 2018. This composition was similar to the US population, which was 50.8% in 2017. During the same

time period, increases for URiM faculty were more modest, increasing from 4.8% to 7.4%. This value stands in contrast to the US population, which was 31.4% URiM in 2017. Examined another way, the number of non-URiM women faculty increased by 13.8 faculty members per year and the number of non-URiM male faculty increased by 10.8 per year between 1970 and 2018. During the same time frame URiM women faculty increased by just 1.2 faculty members per year, whereas URiM men increased by 0.8 faculty members per year.[23] In a separate retrospective study of AACM faculty data from 2007 to 2018, Lu and colleagues[24] confirmed "negligible increases" in URiM representation in academics in that 12-year time span.

A study by Lett and colleagues[25] provides an additional perspective on the issue of URiM underrepresentation in academic dermatology. The investigators compared AAMC faculty data from 1990 and 2016 for 16 medical specialties, including dermatology. The investigators found that blacks and Hispanics were more underrepresented at all faculty levels in 2016 than they were in 1990 across almost all specialties studied, including dermatology, with the exception of black women in obstetrics and gynecology. White women dermatology faculty were noted to be on par with the census in 2016 in this study as they were in the study by Xeireli and colleagues.[23] Looking specifically at the assistant professor level in dermatology, white males were underrepresented, but to a lesser extent than white women, blacks, or Hispanics. Asian males and females were both overrepresented in 2016. At the associate professor level white women were on par with the census in 2016, Asian men and women were overrepresented, and black and Hispanic faculty were underrepresented. At the full professor level white women, blacks, and Hispanics were all underrepresented; Asian women were on par with the census; and Asian and white men were overrepresented. This study provides

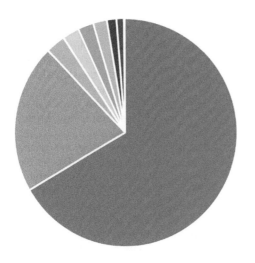

Fig. 2. Racial/ethnic composition of dermatology faculty.

- ■ White 66.6%
- ■ Asian 21.1%
- ■ Black 2.9%
- ■ Hispanic/Latino 2.5%
- ■ Multiple race, Not Hispanic 2.3%
- ■ Multiple race, Hispanic 2.0%
- ■ Unknown 1.4%
- ■ Other 1.1%
- ■ American Indian/Alaska Native 0.1% ■ Native Hawaian 0.0%

additional insight into the plight of URiM faculty, and also points out that although the percentage of white women dermatology faculty is on par with the census overall, this group still faces challenges with parity at the highest academic rank.[25]

Stewart and Lipner[26] also studied diversity among faculty at different ranks. The investigators examined faculty data from 15 top-ranking dermatology departments, including 384 dermatologists, of whom 53.6% were women and 46.4% were men. It was found that 60.7% of women were assistant professors and 17.0% were professors. In contrast, 37.6% of men were assistant professors and 37.6% of men were professors. Women had

fewer publications than men and were less likely to have received National Institutes of Health funding. This study also found that white physicians were more likely to be full professors than nonwhite physicians (31.7% vs 16.7%).[26]

With disparities in the number of women at the rank of full professor, it is not surprising that women are also underrepresented in leadership positions. In the retrospective study by Lu and colleagues[24] from 2007 to 2018, 79.6% of department chairs were men. In a cross-sectional study of all dermatology departments and divisions associated with a residency program, women comprised only 23.5% of chairpersons/division chiefs with 76.5%

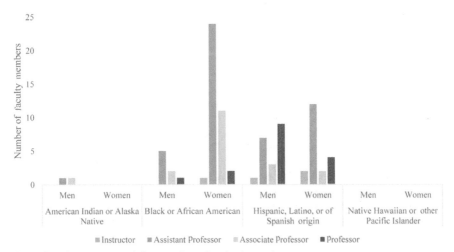

Fig. 3. Number of underrepresented dermatology faculty by rank.

being men.[27] Women have been noted to be under-represented as symposium speakers at the American Academy of Dermatology Annual Meeting.[28]

Barriers to promotion for women and dermatologists underrepresented in medicine

Barriers to academic promotion persist for women and underrepresented physicians. Female faculty face a lack of equity in compensation and support, and are more likely to leave academic medicine compared with their male counterparts.[29] URiM faculty have lower promotional rates and leave full-time faculty positions at a higher rate compared with male and white faculty.[30] Other contributing factors to women and URiM being less likely to progress to senior faculty positions include lack of protected research time, lack of mentorship, fewer opportunities for professional development and networking, and diversity pressures.[31,32] It is important to consider the sometimes subtle and/or unintentional microaggressions and biases that are an all too familiar reality for women and URiM faculty that can influence aspects of the evaluation and promotion process, grant review process, and opportunities for leadership.

URiM faculty share the same clinical, research, and teaching duties as their non-URiM counterparts. However, because patients of color are often sicker and also often seek out physicians of similar racial or ethnic background, the burden of disease of their patient populations may be higher. In addition, URiM physicians often undertake additional work to support the diversity mission of their institution and/or department; they may provide cultural expertise or context to their department by participating in diversity equity and inclusion committees. These physicians may serve as mentors to URiM trainees, who far outnumber the number of URiM faculty within their department. Although URiM faculty are enthusiastic and willing to participate in these diversity initiatives, they do so at the cost of scholarly productivity, which is the primary metric used when evaluating faculty for promotion. Also, URiM physicians take this on while facing microaggressions and macroaggressions themselves. In common terms, these factors, which increase the workload of URiM physicians and decrease productivity by standard academic benchmarks, are often referred to as "cultural tax," the "minority tax" or the "black tax." Efforts in promoting diverse faculty and developing diversity-promoting programs must help to alleviate these additional stressors.

Mentorship is crucial to a successful academic career. Studies have shown that for women and URiM physicians, mentorship plays a critical role in the decision to pursue academic medicine, academic productivity, and job satisfaction.[33,34]

However, women and URiM academicians are less likely to have mentors compared with their peers.[35] The lack of access to mentors can present challenges for people seeking to establish a career in academic medicine.

A diverse faculty may attract a broader patient population, better preparing trainees to care for a wider patient population. Faculty can impart both dermatologic knowledge and cultural awareness to residents and students. Dermatology academic faculty serve as role models to future dermatologists at various stages of training, and through these interactions, they can influence how trainees learn to deliver culturally sensitive and clinically competent care to diverse patients.[23] Greater diversity improves an institution's ability to prepare trainees to care for diverse patients and attend to the needs of diverse patients, in addition to promoting biomedical research that addresses health care disparities and outcomes.[25]

SUMMARY: MOVING TOWARD A MORE INCLUSIVE WORKFORCE

Diversifying dermatology requires an intentional, multifaceted, long-term strategic approach. Ultimately it is the academic departments that most directly bear the responsibility and enjoy the greatest opportunities for shifting the composition of the dermatology workforce over time. The academic departments are the gatekeepers; they control the factors that are prioritized in the initial residency application review. These departments decide which applicants get invited to interview and how they evaluate and rank candidates during the match process, ultimately influencing who matches in the field. And they are responsible for the content of the resident education and the support and mentorship that the residents receive during their training. The academic departments also have the most direct access to the mentor the medical students who are in the pipeline to become dermatology residents.

Ironically, the same academic departments that must embrace and spearhead the diversity charge for the specialty must also confront their own lack of diversity and equity. More information is needed about why URiM dermatologists are not choosing careers in academics, and about barriers to promotion faced by women and URiM faculty members. Faculty retention must be prioritized. At the heart of these issues is the culture of the department. Leadership must be willing to assess and address aspects of their department that may be unwelcoming or unsupportive to women and URiM faculty members.

Of course the responsibility for diversifying the field does not lie only with academic departments. Several investigators have published calls to action, offered roadmaps, or outlined key priority areas to address the workforce.[36,37] Ultimately there are several key areas that need to be targeted, including:

1. Increasing the pipeline of URiM students into college, medical school, and dermatology residency
2. Creating opportunities for early exposure to dermatology, providing URiM medical students with more time to conduct research, increasing clinical exposure to the specialty of dermatology, and supporting academic efforts, ultimately leading to higher likelihood of applying and matching into dermatology
3. Addressing barriers that URiM students face when applying to residency; this includes implementing a holistic review of dermatology residency applicants; considering factors such as lived experiences, distance traveled, and likely contribution to the specialty; as well as grades and scores. It can also include travel stipends for rotations and funding for research projects.[38–40] Implementation of formal mentorship programs, particularly for URiM students and physicians at all points in their education and career, and for women in academics[41–43]
4. Identifying ways to recruit, retain, and promote diverse academic faculty members

Ultimately, addressing these key areas will take a coordinated effort between academic institutions, dermatologic societies, and individuals who are committed to providing excellent care to all patients and to eliminating health disparities.

CLINICS CARE POINTS

- The specialty of dermatology can improve patient outcomes, reduce health disparities and improve patient satisfaction by increasing the diversity of the workforce to inclide more underrepresented and SGM physicians.
- The dermatological subspecialties share the same charge to diversify as the dermatology workforce as a whole does, with issues of lack of diversity in grant funding and organizational leadership in need of particular attention.
- Mentorship is needed to attract, retain and promote women and URiM dermatologists in academics.

ACKNOWLEDGEMENTS

The land upon which we gather and the University of Pennsylvania stands is part of the traditional territory of the Lenni-Lenape, called "Lenapehoking." The Lenape People lived in harmony with one another upon this territory for thousands of years until many were forcibly removed. We acknowledge the Lenni-Lenape as the original people of this land and their continuing relationship with their territory. We affirm the aspiration of the great Lenape Chief Tamanend, that there be harmony between the indigenous people of this land and the descendants of the immigrants to this land, "as long as the rivers and creeks flow, and the sun, moon, and stars shine."

REFERENCES

1. Buster KJ, Stevens EI, Elmets CA. Dermatologic health disparities. Dermatol Clin 2012;30(1):53–9.
2. White RS, Aaronson JA. Obstetric and perinatal racial and ethnic disparities. Curr Opin Anaesthesiol 2022;35(3):260–6.
3. Jang CJ, Lee HC. A review of racial disparities in infant mortality in the US. Child Basel Switz 2022;9(2):257.
4. Center for Disease Control and Prevention. CDC Vital Signs May 2015. Available at: https://www.cdc.gov/vitalsigns/pdf/2015-05-vitalsigns.pdf. Accessed June 16, 2022.
5. Shao K, Hooper J, Feng H. Racial/ethnic health disparities in dermatology in the United States Part 2: disease-specific epidemiology, characteristics, management, and outcomes. J Am Acad Dermatol 2022;87(4):733–44. S0190962222001955.
6. Gorbatenko-Roth K, Prose N, Kundu RV, et al. Assessment of black patients' perception of their dermatology care. JAMA Dermatol 2019;155(10):1129.
7. Gronbeck C, Feng PW, Feng H. Assessment of dermatologist-patient race and ethnicity concordance in the Medicare population. J Am Acad Dermatol 2022;86(3):651–3.
8. Nivet MA. Commentary: diversity 3.0: a necessary systems upgrade. Acad Med 2011;86(12):1487–9.
9. Bodenheimer T, Sinsky C. From triple to quadruple aim: care of the patient requires care of the provider. Ann Fam Med 2014;12(6):573–6.
10. Kirch DG. Increasing diversity and inclusion in medical school to improve the health of all. J Healthc Manag 2013;58(5):311–3.
11. Pandya AG, Alexis AF, Berger TG, et al. Increasing racial and ethnic diversity in dermatology: a call to action. J Am Acad Dermatol 2016;74(3):584–7.
12. National Resident Matching Process. Charting outcomes in the match: senior students of U.S. MD medical schools 2020. Available at: https://www.nrmp.org/wp-content/uploads/2021/08/Charting-Outcomes-in-the-Match-2020_MD-Senior_final.pdf. Accessed June 16, 2022.
13. Association of American Medical Colleges. Physician Specialty Data Report 2020. Available at: https://www.aamc.org/data-reports/workforce/interactive-data/active-physicians-sex-and-specialty-2019. Accessed June 16, 2022.

14. Akoh CC, Shankar S, Strachan DD, et al. Diversifying the dermatology workforce: Physician characteristics vary by race/ethnicity. J Natl Med Assoc 2022. https://doi.org/10.1016/j.jnma.2022.02.011.

15. Mori WS, Gao Y, Linos E, et al. Sexual orientation diversity and specialty choice among graduating allopathic medical students in the United States. JAMA Netw Open 2021;4(9):e2126983.

16. Srivastava R. Gender disparities in income among board-certified dermatologists. Cutis 2021;108(6). https://doi.org/10.12788/cutis.0413.

17. Ashrafzadeh S, Peters GA, Buzney EA, et al. Gender differences in dermatologist practice locations in the United States: A cross-sectional analysis of current gender gaps. Int J Womens Dermatol 2021;7(4):435–40.

18. Sinha S, Lin G, Zubkov M, et al. Geographic distribution and characteristics of the pediatric dermatology workforce in the United States. Pediatr Dermatol 2021;38(6):1523–8.

19. Davies OMT, Benjamin L, Gupta D, et al. Diversity in pediatric dermatology: a report from the Pediatric Dermatology Research Alliance and a call to action. Pediatr Dermatol 2021;38(S2):96–102.

20. Suwattee P, Cham PMH, Abdollahi M, et al. Dermatopathology workforce in the United States: a survey. J Am Acad Dermatol 2011;65(6):1180–5.

21. Feng H, Feng PW, Geronemus RG. Diversity in the US mohs micrographic surgery workforce. Dermatol Surg 2020;46(11):1451–5.

22. Association of American Medical Colleges. U.S. Medical School Faculty by Gender, Race/Ethnicity, Rank, and Department, 2021. Available at: https://www.aamc.org/media/9766/download.

23. Xierali IM, Nivet MA, Pandya AG. US dermatology department faculty diversity trends by sex and underrepresented-in-medicine status, 1970 to 2018. JAMA Dermatol 2020;156(3):280.

24. Lu JD, Tiwana S, Das P, et al. Gender and racial underrepresentation in academic dermatology positions in the United States: A retrospective, cross-sectional study from 2007 to 2018. J Am Acad Dermatol 2020;83(5):1513–6.

25. Lett E, Orji WU, Sebro R. Declining racial and ethnic representation in clinical academic medicine: A longitudinal study of 16 US medical specialties. PLOS ONE 2018;13(11):e0207274.

26. Stewart C, Lipner SR. Gender and race trends in academic rank of dermatologists at top U.S. institutions: a cross-sectional study. Int J Womens Dermatol 2020;6(4):283–5.

27. Shi CR, Olbricht S, Vleugels RA, et al. Sex and leadership in academic dermatology: a nationwide survey. J Am Acad Dermatol 2017;77(4):782–4.

28. Oska S, Touriel R, Partiali B, et al. Women's representation at an academic dermatology conference: trending upwards, but not equal yet. Dermatol Online J 2020;26(3). 13030/qt1pp0073j.

29. Carr PL, Gunn CM, Kaplan SA, et al. Inadequate progress for women in academic medicine: findings from the national faculty study. J Womens Health 2015;24(3):190–9.

30. Fang D, Moy E, Colburn L, et al. Racial and ethnic disparities in faculty promotion in academic medicine. JAMA 2000;284(9):1085–92.

31. Price EG, Powe NR, Kern DE, et al. Improving the diversity climate in academic medicine: faculty perceptions as a catalyst for institutional change. Acad Med J Assoc Am Med Coll 2009;84(1):95–105.

32. Rodríguez JE, Campbell KM, Mouratidis RW. Where are the rest of us? Improving representation of minority faculty in academic medicine. South Med J 2014;107(12):739–44.

33. Dixon G, Kind T, Wright J, et al. Factors that influence the choice of academic pediatrics by underrepresented minorities. Pediatrics 2019;144(2):e20182759.

34. Yehia BR, Cronholm PF, Wilson N, et al. Mentorship and pursuit of academic medicine careers: a mixed methods study of residents from diverse backgrounds. BMC Med Educ 2014;14:26.

35. Beech BM, Calles-Escandon J, Hairston KG, et al. Mentoring programs for underrepresented minority faculty in academic medical centers: a systematic review of the literature. Acad Med J Assoc Am Med Coll 2013;88(4):541–9.

36. Pritchett EN, Pandya AG, Ferguson NN, et al. Diversity in dermatology: roadmap for improvement. J Am Acad Dermatol 2018;79(2):337–41.

37. Granstein RD, Cornelius L, Shinkai K. Diversity in Dermatology-A Call for Action. JAMA Dermatol 2017;153(6):499–500.

38. Luke J, Cornelius L, Lim HW. Dermatology resident selection: shifting toward holistic review? J Am Acad Dermatol 2021;84(4):1208–9.

39. Soliman YS, Rzepecki AK, Guzman AK, et al. Understanding perceived barriers of minority medical students pursuing a career in dermatology. JAMA Dermatol 2019;155(2):252–4.

40. Vasquez R, Jeong H, Florez-Pollack S, et al. What are the barriers faced by under-represented minorities applying to dermatology? A qualitative cross-sectional study of applicants applying to a large dermatology residency program. J Am Acad Dermatol 2020;83(6):1770–3.

41. Saha S, Guiton G, Wimmers PF, et al. Student body racial and ethnic composition and diversity-related outcomes in US medical schools. JAMA 2008;300(10):1135–45.

42. Castiglioni A, Bellini LM, Shea JA. Program directors' views of the importance and prevalence of mentoring in internal medicine residencies. J Gen Intern Med 2004;19(7):779–82.

43. Sambunjak D, Straus SE, Marušić A. Mentoring in academic medicinea systematic review. JAMA 2006;296(9):1103–15.

Diversity, Equity, and Inclusion in Dermatology Residency

Farinoosh Dadrass, MD, MS[a], Sacharitha Bowers, MD[b],
Kanade Shinkai, MD, PhD[c], Kiyanna Williams, MD[d],*

KEYWORDS

- Dermatology • Residency • Diversity • Equity • Inclusion • Education • Apply • Mentor

KEY POINTS

- Dermatology remains one of the least diverse specialties in medicine as it pertains to race and ethnicity. There is less information about other types of diversity and intersectionality in the field.
- Improving diversity, equity, and inclusion (DEI) at the level of the specialty will enhance the workforce and augment the understanding of health-care disparities in the field.
- Improving DEI at the training level will ensure that dermatologists can deliver expert care for diverse populations and address health inequities.
- The successful implementation of DEI initiatives at the residency level has 3 major aims: first, improving the diverse representation of dermatology trainees; second, the development of diverse and inclusive curricula; third, the creation of a more inclusive learning environment and mentorship structures.

INTRODUCTION

Dermatology is currently the fifth least diverse specialty.[1] Despite improvement in diversity efforts, the relative lack of diversity in dermatology thus far has led to significant limitations for individuals within the field, as well as for patients treated by dermatologists, including ongoing health disparities and health inequities in historically minoritized populations.[2–5] There are many different types of diversity including race, gender identity, age, sexual orientation, religion, country of origin, disability, socioeconomic status (SES), housing status, and veteran status. How these various characteristics relate to each other at the individual level is known as intersectionality.[6]

To date, the literature on diversity, equity, and inclusion (DEI) in dermatology is limited and focuses on race, ethnicity, and gender. In 2016, only 3% of dermatologists were Black physicians, not representative of the 12.8% of Black Americans in the general population.[7] Pandya and colleagues[7] described a similar underrepresentation in the Hispanic population, with 4.2% of dermatologists identifying as Hispanic while 16.3% of Americans are Hispanic. A recent study by Mansh and colleagues[8] found 3.7% of dermatologist survey respondents identified as lesbian, gay, bisexual, and transgender and 0.3% identified as transgender. These limited statistics highlight the need for demographic information about the specialty and have prompted many to urge

[a] Loyola University Chicago Stritch School of Medicine, 2160 South 1st Avenue, Maywood, IL 60153, USA;
[b] Division of Dermatology, Department of Internal Medicine, Southern Illinois University, 751 North Rutledge Street, Suite 2300, Springfield, IL 62702, USA; [c] Department of Dermatology, University of California San Francisco, 1701 Divisadero Street, Third Floor, San Francisco, CA 94115, USA; [d] Department of Dermatology, Cleveland Clinic, 9500 Euclid Avenue, Cleveland, OH 44195, USA
* Corresponding author. Cleveland Clinic Department of Dermatology, 2049 E 100th Street, Cleveland, OH 44106.
E-mail address: Kiyanna.williams@gmail.com

Dermatol Clin 41 (2023) 257–263
https://doi.org/10.1016/j.det.2022.10.006

dermatology residency programs to rethink the ways they select their residency applicants.[9]

In this review article, we will identify opportunities for dermatology residency programs to further DEI efforts through improvements in preresidency mentorship, selection of diverse residents, residency curricula, establishing inclusivity in learning environments, and mentorship.

MEDICAL STUDENT PROFESSIONAL IDENTITY FORMATION AND MENTORSHIP

Addressing the lack of racial and ethnic diversity in the dermatology workforce necessitates a critical examination of the barriers to entering dermatology residency training. The percentage of nonwhite students graduating from medical school surpasses the percentage of nonwhite residents in dermatology, suggesting that nonwhite medical students are either not applying into dermatology or not successfully matching into dermatology.[10] Studies suggest reasons that underrepresented minorities (URM) medical students-defined as those belonging to a racial or ethnic group that is underrepresented in the medical field in relation to their numbers in the general population- may not apply include limited interaction with the field both before and while in medical school, less medical school coursework detailing diseases in patients with skin of color (SOC), less engagement with the community from dermatologists, and the increasing competitiveness of matching into dermatology.[11] A cross-sectional study by Vasquez and colleagues [12]identified 6 themes that serve as barriers for URM students applying to dermatology: lack of equitable resources, lack of support, financial constraints, lack of group identity, mentorship, and pipeline or enrichment programs.

Gap year programs, such as predoctoral research fellowships, have become common with approximately half of dermatology applicants completing one.[13] In 2020, the average number of abstracts, presentations, and publications for senior US MD, US DO, and non-US IMG students who matched into dermatology were 19.0, 7.3, and 34.8, respectively.[14–16] Despite an increasing number of publications among matched candidates, there is no data to suggest that a research fellowship increases the likelihood of matching into dermatology. Although research years can provide valuable experiences, publications, and opportunities for letters of recommendation, they can be costly due to relocation and living expenses. Many of these gap years are unpaid, which may preclude applicants with low SES.[17] The low authentic value of this gap year is suggested by students' statements that they would not have pursued a gap research year if they were not applying to a competitive residency.

Currently, there are several collaborative efforts among specialty groups in dermatology that have focused on DEI to transform dermatology into a specialty that is more diverse, inclusive, culturally competent, and equitable.[18] DEI initiatives in dermatology and other specialties focused on medical students include virtual electives and specialty career fairs for URM students, increasing departmental Grand Rounds content featuring DEI topics, and preinterview meetings with URM applicants.[19–21] Additional pipeline and community initiatives, early exposure to dermatology through the introduction of educational content similar to the AAD Skin of Color Graduate Medical Education Series, and longitudinal mentoring in both structured (eg, organizations, societies, programs) and unstructured formats, may also reduce barriers to applying to dermatology.

SELECTING DIVERSE DERMATOLOGY RESIDENTS

Improving the diversity of the workforce must begin with the selection of diverse dermatology residents. Data have shown that URM trainees match into dermatology at lower rates despite similar numbers of away rotations and interviews.[22] One study examining the surgical residency application process addressed the concept of disqualification by "culture fit," where faculty may deem an applicant to be qualified for the position but not be a good "fit" for the program.[22] However, dermatology as a specialty has the potential to experience greater growth from diverse perspectives and mindsets if programs searched for applicants who would instead be a "culture add."[23] Following the requirement of Implicit Association Tests (IATs) for medical school admissions committee members, Capers IV and colleagues[24] reported an increase in the diversity of their matriculated applicants despite the diversity of their accepted applicants remaining relatively constant. Some have recommended deemphasis on application components subject to bias including honors grading and AOA status.[22]

Holistic review has been proposed as one solution to achieve better representation in dermatology residency selection. The process highlights assessment of attributes that are key to being a physician and align with organizational values, such as humanism, empathy, resilience, growth mindset, and interpersonal skills. The 2021 National Resident Matching Program Program Director Survey has shown positive trends that may reflect the benefits of holistic review.[25] This includes improved value of humanism and cultural competency, such as Gold Humanism Honor Society membership and fluency in the language of the patient population served, with reduced emphasis on the United States Medical Licensing Exam (USMLE) Step 1 and USMLE Step 2 scores.[25,26]

In the 2021 to 2022 application cycle, the new Electronic Residency Application Service (ERAS) Supplemental Application pilot program was created to standardize and highlight additional components of an application for holistic review while programs receive an increasing number of applications.[27,28] The supplemental application allows students to optionally send 3 preference signals, which indicate their particular interest in receiving an interview from that program, as well to convey geographic preferences. Additionally, as of January 26, 2022, USMLE Step 1 scores will now be reported on a pass or fail outcome.

To mitigate bias in the residency selection process, it is recommended that residency selection committees include individuals from diverse backgrounds. Additionally, they should all be required to complete IATs and DEI training, as well as use the AAMC Diversity and Inclusion Toolkit Resources. It remains unclear how residency programs will choose to assess applications moving forward without a numerical USMLE Step 1 score. One opportunity is to use ERAS preference signaling to enhance equity in the application process by offering additional preference signals to URM students and applicants without home dermatology programs but this option has not yet been made available.

RESIDENCY: CURRICULUM

An important aspect of improving DEI in dermatology is addressing known gaps in the dermatology residency curriculum to enable dermatologists to provide expert care to all patients, prevent clinician bias, and also to address known health disparities in patients with SOC.[29] Duke University and the University of Pennsylvania recently created Diversity and Community Engagement dermatology residency positions reserved for those interested in working with underserved populations and patients with SOC. An additional gap in residency curriculum is SGM content. A web-based survey found that most curricular content centered around HIV/AIDS, with little emphasis on other dermatologic conditions seen in SGM individuals.[30] To address gaps in SOC and SGM curriculum, the AAD released a Skin of Color Graduate Medical Education series

in Spring 2022 and a Sexual and Gender Diverse Dermatology module within the AAD Basic Derm Curriculum. Furthermore, individual dermatology residency programs have started to create their own SOC and/or SGM curricula as well as curricula on Social Determinants of Health.[31–33] There have been calls to action for the implementation of standardized guidelines and a curriculum to improve dermatologic knowledge and care for individuals with disabilities.[34,35]

Because the AAD and individual dermatology residency programs begin to create these resources, it is important to consider how this curriculum can be standardized and taught to all dermatology residents as well as those already board-certified. Rigorous, inclusive research will also be crucial to inform the inclusion of recommendations for high-value care for diverse patients in trainee education.

RESIDENCY: CREATING AN INCLUSIVE LEARNING ENVIRONMENT IN DERMATOLOGY RESIDENCY PROGRAMS

Creating a culture of inclusion is paramount to the overall success and well-being of a diverse residency program. However, there are several factors that challenge this aim including overt racism, discriminatory implicit bias, lack of structured SOC training, and lack of cultural competence. Although overt forms of discriminatory behavior have known impacts on an individual's health and well-being, recent research has focused more on less overt forms of discrimination and bias termed microaggressions, which may be supplanting more pronounced acts of bias such that racism is perpetuated in more insidious and seemingly socially acceptable, but no less harmful, ways.[36–38]

Medical students and residents who experience these forms of bias are more likely to report associated symptoms of burnout, depression, and suicidal thoughts.[39–41] A recent study showed that 61% of medical student respondents reported experiencing at least one microaggression weekly. These medical students were more likely to consider medical school transfer and withdrawal, and more likely to think microaggressions were a normal part of medical school culture.[42] These experiences can further lead to minority status stress, racial battle fatigue, feelings of invisibility, isolation, exclusion, and loneliness.[43,44] Furthermore, discrimination has shown to influence job satisfaction and turnover with physicians who experience discrimination reporting lower job satisfaction and being more likely to contemplate career change than physicians without these experiences.[45]

Several studies have examined trainings and interventions to address microaggressions in 5 domains: establishing a supportive culture, addressing microaggressions, supporting targets of microaggressions, discriminatory requests, and institutional recommendations.[46] Literature suggests to establish a supportive culture: it is important that health-care organizations create a system for reporting microaggressions and support health-care professionals to receive training on responding to these types of discrimination.[47] Several studies have found health-care professionals need and want to learn how to address microaggressions.[48,49] Many articles suggest the first step to battling microaggressions is to first identify their occurrence and bring them to the forefront of everyone's awareness as a way to remove the oppressive power of the event over the marginalized individual.[50]

It is important to support the targets of microaggressions, which can be done by debriefing, setting limits with patients, seeking support from other health-care workers, and reporting of the incident.[47,51–53] Furthermore, discriminatory requests made by patients asking for a different health-care provider should also be addressed.

It is imperative that dermatology become a specialty where underrepresented minorities see themselves as members, as leaders. Diversifying the workforce is the most critical step to fostering inclusivity by proving by example the importance of representation and inclusion. It is paramount to the success of diversity and inclusion efforts that stakeholders from every level of leadership be invested and involvement of a more diverse leadership team should be emphasized to ensure a safe and inclusive learning environment.

IMPROVING THE FUTURE LEADERSHIP OF DERMATOLOGY THROUGH INTENTIONAL MENTORSHIP

One of the previously identified barriers to applying to dermatology that URM students face is lack of mentorship.[12] Reasons for the limited availability of race-concordant dermatology mentors are 2-fold. The first is the small number of URM faculty in academic dermatology as well as dermatology in general.[7,54] Second, the concept of minority or cultural taxation often leads to URM faculty spending more of their time toward DEI efforts rather than focusing on other career milestones and advancement metrics, which traditionally lead to promotion and tenure.[55,56] For these reasons, in addition to the recruitment and retention of URM faculty, race-discordant mentorship and allyship in diversity efforts is essential.

In race-discordant mentorship dyads, it is important for mentors to recognize that a special skillset is needed to mentor URM trainees beyond basic mentoring skills. For mentors to understand URM trainees' background and how to best support them, self-education on opportunities and resources available to URM trainees is crucial. Additional key principles for mentoring URM trainees include understanding stereotype threat, explicit support, and an openness and welcoming to debrief on issues regarding inclusivity and dealing with microaggressions.[47,57] Finally, mentors should use their existing professional and personal networks to introduce URM mentees to others, including racially concordant mentors, thus enhancing visibility within the field. They would further be encouraged to strengthen and broaden his/her network to connect with more URM faculty that can be introduced to their mentees. Mentors should also know what funding, clinical, and research opportunities are uniquely available to URM students at local and national levels in order to actively promote them.

There are many different forms of mentorship and mentor roles, and often mentees may require more than one mentor.[58] Reasons for mentorship failure range from limited access to mentors, differing communication styles, lack of clear expectations, assigned mentor-mentee pairs that feel "forced," and racial, ethnic, and gender differences that may be difficult to navigate.[59,60] Further faculty development can be found in the AAD Skin of Color Graduate Medical Education Series module entitled "Mentoring underrepresented minority dermatologists and trainees: Best practices for success." A final concept worth highlighting is the notion of "developing talent–not sorting it" by Dhaliwal and colleagues,[61] which challenges faculty to have a growth mindset in developing trainees to achieve their fullest potential.

Mentorship of URM physicians is critical and has shown to play a key role in the decision to pursue academic medicine, academic productivity, and job satisfaction.[62,63] It is important that faculty receive protected time to participate in professional development opportunities because this has been shown to improve recruitment and retention while also offering an additional opportunity for junior faculty to find mentors.

SUMMARY

To date, DEI initiatives within dermatology have provided solutions for applicants to be successful in the current system. However, additional steps are needed to change the system itself to be more inclusive, and to ensure that inclusiveness can be operationalized at all levels of the specialty. A diverse workforce begins with diverse trainees who are supported to learn to provide expert care to all patients and address health disparities. Inclusive efforts and intentional mentorship, in time, will develop, retain, and empower future diverse leaders of dermatology to uphold a system that provides excellent care for all.

CLINICS CARE POINTS

- Improving DEI in dermatology will require diversifying our workforce through resident selection processes and structured mentorship and sponsorship or URM trainees.

- Improving DEI will lead to decreased healthcare disparities and increase in culturally competent care Creating more inclusive learning environments will aid in the development of culturally competent physicians who can then provide the highest quality care to patients.

DISCLOSURE

The authors have no conflicts of interest or funding sources to disclose.

REFERENCES

1. Lopez S, Lourido JO, Lim HW, et al. The call to action to increase racial and ethnic diversity in dermatology: A retrospective, cross-sectional study to monitor progress. J Am Acad Dermatol 2022;86(3):e121–3.
2. Zheng YJ, Ho C, Lazar A, et al. Poor melanoma outcomes and survival in Asian American and Pacific Islander patients. J Am Acad Dermatol 2021;84(6):1725–7.
3. Koblinski JE, Maykowski P, Zeitouni NC. Disparities in melanoma stage at diagnosis in Arizona: a 10-year Arizona Cancer Registry study. J Am Acad Dermatol 2021;84(6):1776–9.
4. Qian Y, Johannet P, Sawyers A, et al. The ongoing racial disparities in melanoma: an analysis of the Surveillance, Epidemiology, and End Results database (1975-2016). J Am Acad Dermatol 2021;84(6):1585–93.
5. Cortez JL, Vasquez J, Wei ML. The impact of demographics, socioeconomics, and health care access on melanoma outcomes. J Am Acad Dermatol 2021;84(6):1677–83.
6. Bowleg L. The problem with the phrase women and minorities: intersectionality-an important theoretical framework for public health. Am J Public Health 2012;102(7):1267–73.
7. Pandya AG, Alexis AF, Berger TG, et al. Increasing racial and ethnic diversity in dermatology: a call to action. J Am Acad Dermatol 2016;74(3):584–7.
8. Mansh MD, Dommasch E, Peebles JK, et al. Lesbian, gay, bisexual, and transgender identity and disclosure among dermatologists in the US. JAMA Dermatol 2021;157(12):1512–4.
9. Chen A, Shinkai K. Rethinking how we select dermatology applicants-turning the tide. JAMA Dermatol 2017;153(3):259–60.
10. Van Voorhees AS, Enos CW. Diversity in dermatology residency programs. J Investig Dermatol Symp Proc 2017;18(2):S46–9.
11. Bae G., Qiu M., Reese E., et al., Changes in Sex and Ethnic Diversity in Dermatology Residents Over Multiple Decades, JAMA Dermatol, 152 (1), 2016, 92-94.
12. Vasquez R, Jeong H, Florez-Pollack S, et al. What are the barriers faced by under-represented minorities applying to dermatology? A qualitative cross-sectional study of applicants applying to a large dermatology residency program. J Am Acad Dermatol 2020;83(6):1770–3.
13. Rodriguez R, Siller A Jr, Pandya AG, et al. Implications of increasing publication trends in dermatology on individuals from disadvantaged backgrounds and those without a home dermatology program. J Am Acad Dermatol 2021;84(2):e109–10.
14. Charting outcomes in the match: senior students of U.S. medical schools. In: National resident matching program. 2020. Available at: https://www.nrmp.org/wp-content/uploads/2021/08/Charting-Outcomes-in-the-Match-2020_MD-Senior_final.pdf 2020. Accessed May 7, 2022.
15. Charting outcomes in the match: senior students of U.S. DO medical schools. In: National resident matching program. 2020. Available at: https://www.nrmp.org/wp-content/uploads/2021/08/Charting-Outcomes-in-the-Match-2020_DO-Senior_final.pdf 2020. Accessed May 7, 2022.
16. Charting outcomes in the match: international medical graduates. In: National resident matching program. 2020. Available at: https://www.nrmp.org/wp-content/uploads/2021/08/Charting-Outcomes-in-the-Match-2020_IMG_final.pdf 2020. Accessed May 7, 2022.
17. Runge M, Jairath NK, Renati S, et al. Pursuit of a research year or dual degree by dermatology residency applicants: a cross-sectional study. Cutis 2022;109(1):E12–3.
18. Desai SR, Khanna R, Glass D, et al. Embracing diversity in dermatology: Creation of a culture of equity and inclusion in dermatology. Int J Womens Dermatol 2021;7(4):378–82.
19. Harpe JM, Safdieh JE, Broner S, et al. The development of a diversity, equity, and inclusion committee

in a neurology department and residency program. J Neurol Sci 2021;428:117572.

20. Ojo E, Hairston D. Recruiting Underrepresented Minority Students into Psychiatry Residency: a Virtual Diversity Initiative. Acad Psychiatry 2021;45(4): 440–4.

21. Mendiola M, Modest AM, Huang GC. Striving for diversity: national survey of OB-GYN program directors reporting residency recruitment strategies for underrepresented minorities. J Surg Educ 2021; 78(5):1476–82.

22. Costello CM, Harvey JA, Besch-Stokes JG, et al. The role of race and ethnicity in the dermatology applicant match process. J Natl Med Assoc 2022; 113(6):666–70.

23. Modest JM, Cruz AI Jr, Daniels AH, et al. Applicant fit and diversity in the orthopaedic surgery residency selection process: defining and melding to create a more diverse and stronger residency program. JB JS Open Access 2020;5(4):e20.00074.

24. Capers Q 4th, Clinchot D, McDougle L, et al. Implicit racial bias in medical school admissions. Acad Med 2017;92(3):365–9.

25. Results of the 2021 NRMP program director survey. In: National resident matching program. 2021. Available at: https://www.nrmp.org/wp-content/uploads/2021/11/2021-PD-Survey-Report-for-WWW.pdf 2021. Accessed May 7, 2022.

26. Results of the 2014 NRMP program director survey. In: National resident matching program. 2014. Available at: https://www.nrmp.org/wp-content/uploads/2021/07/PD-Survey-Report-2014.pdf 2014. Accessed May 7, 2022.

27. AAMC supplemental ERAS® application: key findings from the 2022 application cycle. In: AAMC. 2022. Available at: https://www.aamc.org/media/58891/download 2022. Accessed May 8, 2022.

28. Weiner S. Everything you need to know about the supplemental ERAS® application. In: AAMC. 2021. Available at: https://www.aamc.org/news-insights/everything-you-need-know-about-supplemental-eras-application 2021. Accessed May 8, 2022.

29. Buster K, Ezenwa E. Health disparities and skin cancer in people of color. In: Practical dermatology. 2019. Available at: https://practicaldermatology.com/articles/2019-apr/health-disparities-and-skin-cancer-in-people-of-color 2019. Accessed May 8, 2022.

30. Jia JL, Nord KM, Sarin KY, et al. Sexual and gender minority curricula within US dermatology residency programs. JAMA Dermatol 2020;156(5):593–4.

31. Mhlaba JM, Pontes DS, Patterson SS, et al. Evaluation of a skin of color curriculum for dermatology residents. J Drugs Dermatol 2021;20(7):786–9.

32. Jia JL, Gordon JS, Lester JC, et al. Integrating skin of color and sexual and gender minority content into dermatology residency curricula: A prospective program initiative. J Am Acad Dermatol 2022;86(5): 1119–20.

33. Barrett DL, Supapannachart KJ, Caleon RL, et al. Interactive session for residents and medical students on dermatologic care for lesbian, gay, bisexual, transgender, and queer patients. MedEd-PORTAL 2021;17:11148.

34. Nassim JS, Watson AJ, Tan JK. Achieving equitable care for people with disabilities: considerations for the dermatologist. JAMA Dermatol 2020;156(11): 1173–5.

35. Dawson J, Smogorzewski J. Demystifying disability assessments for dermatologists-a call to action. JAMA Dermatol 2021;157(8):903–4.

36. Pierce CM, Carew JV, Pierce-Gonzales D, et al. An experiment in racism: TV commercials. Education Urban Soc 1997;10:61–87.

37. Fields KE. Racecraft the soul of inequality in American Life. London: Verso; 2012.

38. Benjamin R. Innovating inequity: if race is a technology, postracialism is the genius bar. Ethnic Racial Stud 2016;39(13):2227–34.

39. Chisholm LP, Jackson KR, Davidson HA, et al. Evaluation of racial microaggressions experienced during medical school training and the effect on medical student education and burnout: a validation study. J Natl Med Assoc 2020;113(3). S0027-9684(20)30428-4.

40. Hu YY, Ellis RJ, Hewitt DB, et al. Discrimination, abuse, harassment, and burnout in surgical residency training. N Engl J Med 2019;381:1741–52.

41. Dyrbye LN, Thomas MR, Eacker A, et al. Race, ethnicity, and medical student well-being in the United States. Arch Intern Med 2007;167(19):2103–9.

42. Anderson N, Lett E, Asabor EN, et al. The association of microaggressions with depressive symptoms and institutional satisfaction among a national cohort of medical students. J Gen Intern Med 2022;37(2): 298–307.

43. Acholonu RG, Oyeku SO. Addressing microaggressions in the healthcare workforce-a path toward achieving equity and inclusion. JAMA Netw Open 2020;3(11):3E2021770.

44. O'Keefe VM, Wingate LR, Cole AB, et al. Seemingly harmless racial communications are not so harmless: racial microaggressions lead to suicidal ideation by way of depressive symptoms. Suicide Life Threat Behav 2015;45:567–76.

45. Nunez-Smith M, Pilgrim N, Wynia M, et al. Health care workplace discrimination and physician turnover. J Intl Med Assoc 2009;101(12):1274–82.

46. Wittkower LD, Bryan JL, Ashgar-Ali AA. A scoping review of recommendations and training to respond to patient microaggressions. Acad Psych 2021; 46(5):627–39.

47. Wheeler DJ, Zapata J, Davis D, et al. Twelve tips for responding to microaggressions and overt

discrimination: when the patient offends the learner. Med Teach 2019;41(10):1112–7.

48. Baby M, Swain N, Gale C. Healthcare managers' perceptions of patient perpetrated aggression and prevention strategies: a cross sectional survey. Issues Ment Health Nurs 2016;37(7):507–16.

49. Hills DJ, Joyce CM, Humphreys JS. Prevalence and prevention of workplace aggression in Australian clinical medical practice. Aust Health Rev 2011; 35(3):253–61.

50. Sue DW, Capodilupo CM, Torino GC, et al. Racial microaggressions in everyday life: implications for clinical practice. Am Psychol 2007;62(4):271–86.

51. Brophy JT, Keith MM, Hurley M. Assaulted and unheard: violence against healthcare staff. New Solut 2017;27(4):1–26.

52. Paul-Emile K, Critchfield JM, Wheeler M, et al. Addressing patient bias toward health care workers: recommendations for medical centers. Ann Int Med 2020;173(6):468–73.

53. Thurber A, DiAngelo R. Microaggressions intervening in three acts. J Ethn Cult Divers Soc Work 2018;27(1):17–27.

54. Bae G, Qiu M, Reese E, et al. Changes in sex and ethnic diversity in dermatology residents over multiple decades. JAMA Dermatol 2016;152(1):92–4.

55. Okoye GA. Supporting underrepresented minority women in academic dermatology. Int J Womens Dermatol 2019;6(1):57–60.

56. Williams K, Shinkai K. The leaky pipeline: a narrative review of diversity in dermatology. Cutis 2022; 109(1):27–31.

57. Negbenebor NA. Advice for applying to dermatology as an applicant of color: keep going. Cutis 2021;107(1):E15–6.

58. 4 phases of mentoring relationships. In: EDUCAUSE. Available at: https://www.educause.edu/-/media/files/wiki-import/2014infosecurityguide/mentoring-toolkit/siguccsmentorguidepdf. Accessed May 3, 2022.

59. Soliman YS, Rzepecki AK, Guzman AK, et al. Understanding Perceived Barriers of Minority Medical Students Pursuing a Career in Dermatology. JAMA Dermatol 2019;155(2):252–4.

60. Sambunjak D, Straus SE, Marusic A. A systematic review of qualitative research on the meaning and characteristics of mentoring in academic medicine. J Gen Intern Med 2010;25(1):72–8.

61. Dhaliwal G, Hauer KE. Excellence in medical training: developing talent-not sorting it. Perspect Med Educ 2021;10(6):356–61.

62. Beech BM, Calles-Escandon J, Hairston KC, et al. Mentoring programs for underrepresented minority faculty in academic medical center: a systematic review of the literature. Acad Med 2013;88(4):541–9.

63. Daley S, Wingard DL, Reznik V. Improving the retention of underrepresented minority faculty in academic medicine. J Natl Med Assoc 2006;98(9): 1435–40.

Gender Equity in Medicine and Dermatology in the United States
The Long Road Traveled and the Journey ahead

Janell M. Tully, BS[a,b], Jenny E. Murase, MD[a,c,1], Jane M. Grant-Kels, MD[d,e,1], Dedee F. Murrell, MA, BMBCh, MD, FRCP[f,*,1]

KEYWORDS

- Gender • Gender equity • Academic medicine • Diversity • Leadership • Women in medicine
- Mentorship • Authorship

KEY POINTS

- Women account for roughly half of dermatology resident trainees and academic faculty.
- Women in academic medicine are significantly more likely to hold junior titles and remain underrepresented as senior faculty, in research and leadership positions.
- The limited number of women in academic leadership results in a dearth of role models for younger women to identify with, which may, in turn, leave them feeling unsupported as they navigate their career and day-to-day responsibilities and more likely to leave academic medicine.
- Gender bias plays a critical role in the development and persistence of gender inequity within academic medicine.

INTRODUCTION

Gender refers to a social construct, based on sex assigned at birth, that society often uses to establish expectations of how individuals should behave and what roles they are apt to fulfill.[1] For example, women are traditionally expected to be caring homemakers, whereas men are to be assertive and work outside of the home.[2] Women pursuing fruitful careers as physicians, inconsistent with traditional gender expectations, can have meaningful career implications for women that men do not otherwise encounter.

Although men and women graduate from medical training at similar rates, gender gaps in leadership, research publications, and compensation persist. Gender bias disproportionately impacts women with children early in their careers, contributing to the development and persistence of gender inequity in academia.[3–5]

Before 1970, few women were granted entrance into medical school. By 1970 women accounted for 11% of medical students and less than 8% of academic medicine faculty in the United States.[6] In 1972 Congress passed Title IX, a landmark law for gender equality by prohibiting federally funded

a Department of Dermatology, University of California, San Francisco, 1701 Divisadero Street, San Francisco, CA 94115, USA; b University of Arizona College of Medicine – Phoenix, 475 N 5th St, Phoenix, AZ 85004, USA; c Department of Dermatology, Palo Alto Foundation Medical Group, 701 East El Camino Real, Mountain View, CA 94040, USA; d Department of Dermatology, University of Connecticut School of Medicine, UCONN Health, 21 South Road, Farmington, CT 06032, USA; e Department of Dermatology, University of Florida College of Medicine, 4037 NW 86th Terrace, 4th Floor, Gainesville, FL 32606, USA; f Department of Dermatology, St. George Hospital, University of New South Wales, 27 Belgrave St, Kogarah, NSW 2217, Australia
1 Co-senior authorship.
* Corresponding author.
E-mail address: d.murrell@unsw.edu.au

Dermatol Clin 41 (2023) 265–278
https://doi.org/10.1016/j.det.2022.08.007

education programs from excluding individuals based on sex or gender identity.[7] Simultaneously, the number of women applying to and entering medical school rose rapidly.[8] Approximately 40 years later, women graduate from medical school at similar rates to men.[9] Similarly, the proportion of women in dermatology also increased substantially, and women represented 60% of residents and more than half of academic faculty in 2017.[10] As of February 2022, it was reported that 53% of practicing dermatologists in the United States are women.[11] Despite this growth, there remains an unequivocal gender imbalance within academic medicine.

Given the historical imbalances seen throughout academic medicine and the considerable impact on women's careers,[12,13] we assessed the current status of gender equity among women in academic medicine with a particular focus on dermatology. Herein, we explore trends in the representation of women in academic leadership and evaluate the roles of mentorship, motherhood, and gender bias on gender equity. Moreover, we used peer-reviewed publications to offer constructive solutions for addressing gender inequities that persist in academic medicine today.

Gender Differences in Academic Leadership

The percentage of women among full-time dermatology faculty has substantially increased in the United States from less than 11% in 1970% to 51% in 2018.[10] For the first time in 2017, the proportion of full-time female dermatology faculty surpassed the proportion of full-time male faculty, reflecting the percentage of women in medicine and dermatology[10]

On the surface, this equal representation of women in dermatology continues to be seen among assistant professors with women accounting for 56% of all assistant professors in academic medicine.[14] However, only 17% of full-time women academic dermatologists hold the title of full professor. In contrast, more than one-third of full-time men's academic faculty account for over 65% of all full dermatology professors.[15]

Despite the increase of female professors since the 1970s, less than 39% of program directors, 19% of departmental chairs, and roughly 18% of all deans across academic medicine were women in 2019.[16,17] As seen with the representation of women as academic professors, one study found significant improvements in gender disparity among junior dean positions (eg, assistant deans), but little change at the level of vice and executive dean.[18] In 2018, The American Association of Medical Colleges (AAMC) reported

similar findings, where women continued to account for more than half of assistant deans but only one-third of senior associate and vice deans across US medical schools.[9] The proportion of women deans also varies greatly by office. Women are well represented as deans in the offices of diversity, equity, and inclusion, but remain greatly underrepresented in clinical and research departments (**Table 1**).[19]

Women accounted for 28% of dermatology department chairs in 2019, which was 9% higher than the proportion of women department chairs across academic medicine.[17] However, given that dermatology has a higher percentage of women faculty as compared with all academic faculty (52% vs 42%, respectively),[17] the representation of women chairpersons in dermatology is reflective of the general underrepresentation of women throughout academic medicine. Although this may be slowly changing as the percentage of women dermatology chairpersons increased to 33% in a single year.[20]

In 2020, women accounted for 31% of dermatology division chiefs.[20] In addition to being appointed as a chair or chief at similar ages (46 years) more than half of men and women chairs are actively engaged in research.[21,22] Interestingly, despite the overall high annual turnover rate of chairpersons, women, on average, leave their position 6 years earlier than men.[21]

Women have represented roughly 50% of dermatology program directors since 2016,[17,23] a notable increase from 28% in 2009.[24] However, when compared with the percentage of all female dermatology faculty, this proportion paralleled the underrepresentation of women program directors throughout academic medicine.[17] When evaluating the gender distribution of program directors and chairpersons within a single program, one study found that although 33% of dermatology programs had both a male chair and male program director, no program had two females in these roles concurrently.[23]

Gender Differences in Compensation in Academic Medicine

Women in academic medicine are not only underrepresented among leadership positions, but they are also paid significantly less than their male counterparts. In a January 2020 call to action, the AAMC issued a statement acknowledging that despite equal effort, experience, training, and professional rank, women were unfairly compensated across multiple domains as compared with their male peers.[25,26] Women, on average, have lower starting salaries, receive

Table 1
The proportion of female deans by office and rank

Office	Assistant Deans (% Female)	Associate Deans (% Female)	Senior Associate/ Vice Deans (% Female)
Diversity, Equity, and Inclusion	56%	68%	57%
Research	34%	39%	26%
Clinical/Health Affairs	40%	33%	15%

Notes: The percentage of female deans across academic offices and by rank.[18]

lower bonuses, and are penalized (eg, perceived as more demanding and less desirable to work with) more frequently than men when negotiating pay.[27–29]

After controlling for provider and practice characteristics as well as the patient volume between 1992 and 2002, female dermatologists made roughly $80,000 (28%) less than their male colleagues,[30] which remained unchanged over 15 years later.[31] A more recent study among academic physicians, found that from 2013 to 2018, women experienced a larger increase in salary growth compared with men (20% vs 9%, respectively), resulting in roughly a $30,000 reduction in the $80,000 gap in pay seen in 2013.[32] These findings offer a promising outlook that the pay gap may be, albeit slowly, narrowing within academic medicine.

Multiple studies have attempted to elucidate what variables play a role in the gender salary gap. Three common themes across studies of gender disparity in academic dermatology are that: (1) women are younger, (2) work fewer hours, and (3) are less well represented at levels of leadership than men. When controlling for these, among other covariates, the pay gap persists.[31,33,34] One study found that after adjusting for seniority and leadership rank, male dermatologists continued to make 17% more than females.[34] Conversely, despite finding a significant discrepancy in pay between men and women after adjusting for academic rank and promotion, one study found that the gender difference was no longer significant after adjusting for full-time working status.[35] These findings, however, contrast with prior studies. After running a thousand Monte Carlo simulated data sets, a statistical model used to predict the likelihood of a particular outcome,[36] male dermatologists' salaries remained significantly higher than their female peers, suggesting that difference in salary cannot be explained by the amount of time spent working.[34] Furthermore, one study reported that although hours worked and patient volume were both significant predictors of annual income, men still had significantly

higher wages after controlling for both variables.[31] If salaries were standardized rather than negotiated, this would create an equal framework for women.

Gender Differences in Private Practice

Although workforce challenges in academic settings likely differ from those in private practice,[37] most published studies on gender equity among dermatologists focus on academic medicine. Of the studies that include private practices in their analyses of gender differences, they often control for practice type (eg, academic, group, or private practice) making it difficult to ascertain gender differences in non-academic settings.[30,31,37,38] Thus, the representation of women among private practice leadership, financial compensation, and whether the organizational structure of private practice contributes to gender inequity need to be explored in the future.[3,10]

Gender Differences in Research Publications

A gender gap persists despite significant increases in the representation of women authors in peer-reviewed journals since the 1970s.[6] From 1976 to 2006, there was a 4-fold increase in the number of female first authors and a 5-fold increase in female senior authors (**Fig. 1**).[6] Since 2006, the percentage of female first authors in top-scoring dermatology journals reached roughly 50% and remained relatively stable through 2019.[39,40] One dermatology journal, *Contact Dermatitis*, reported an even greater increase in female first authors, increasing from 37% in 1992% to 66% in 2019.[41] This equates to an average annual percentage increase of 3%, almost double the increase seen over the past 15 years across top dermatology journals,[40] however, this is still a significant reduction from the 10% average annual increase seen between 1976 and 2006.[6]

Although the percentage of first female authors has reached more equitable representation, females continued to account for one-third of senior authors between 2008 and 2017 across top-

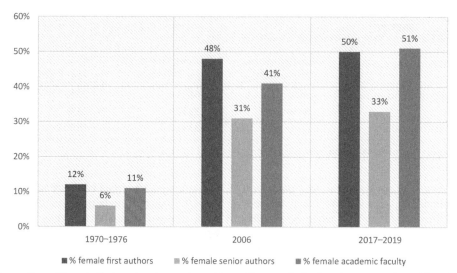

Fig. 1. Proportion of female first and senior authors. Notes: The graph depicts the proportion of female first and senior authors in comparison to the percentage of female faculty from the 1970s through 2019.[6,10,39,40]

scoring dermatology journals (see **Fig. 1**).[40] The annual increase in female senior authors over the past 15 years was considerably smaller than the rapid annual rise seen between 1976 and 2006 (3% vs 14%, respectively).[6,40] Again, *Contact Dermatitis* stood out with an increase of female senior authors from 27% in 1992% to 61% in 2019, representing an average annual percentage change of approximately 5%.[41] (**Fig. 1**).

Notably, the *International Journal of Women's Dermatology* (IJWD) has maintained a high degree of female authorship since its first publication in 2015 with 96% of articles having at least one female author.[42] However, among high-impact general medicine journals, the overall representation of females as first authors is much lower, ranging from 20% to 45% between 2009 and 2014.[43] Moreover, some general medical journals have either showed stagnant growth or a decline in female authorship over the past 50 years.[43] In leading medical education journals, however, female first authorship increased from 7% in 1970 to nearly 54% in 2019 and senior authorship increased from less than 10% to 46%.[44]

Considerable progress has been made over the past five decades among women with first authorship publications. Additional research shows that women continue to have a large amount of ground to cover across peer-reviewed journals to achieve gender equity. First, men are more likely to have 3 or more publications, whereas women are more likely to have a single publication in a peer-reviewed dermatology journal.[40] Additionally, although men account for 53% of authors, they hold 57% of all authorships and are more likely to be a senior author than women.[40]

Men are two times more likely to be invited to submit their work in journals,[45] and in cases where men and women contribute equally to a publication, men are significantly more likely to have their name printed first in the publication, regardless of alphabetical order.[46] Men are also more likely to publish in prestigious journals, especially as senior authors.[47] Furthermore, when looking at the gender of corresponding authors, one group found that male corresponding authors are significantly more likely than their female counterparts to be published in prestigious journals.[48]

The proportion of women represented as authors in peer-reviewed journals has been found to be highly variable,[6,40,43,47] ranging from less than 33% to over 53% in leading dermatology journals.[40] Not all studies have found significant gender differences in authorship between journals, including two studies evaluating a few select general dermatology journals with significant overlap of journals between studies.[6,40] Of the 3 general dermatology journals evaluated in each study, both included the *Journal of the American Academy of Dermatology* (JAAD) and the *Journal of Investigate Dermatology* (JID). Therefore, the lack of variation between journals seen in these two studies is likely more representative of the overlapping, small sample size of high-impact journals rather than the overall lack of variability between all journals. Notably, however, is that female first authorship is significantly associated with having a female senior author on the same publication.[6,40,44,49]

Impact of Research Productivity on Publications

The literature covers a breadth of reasons to elucidate why women have significantly lower research productivity than men. Women faculty may spend less time on research tasks than men, especially early in their career.[50–52] Some have attributed this to women with children working fewer hours.[38,53,54] Moreover, women are more likely to take on educator roles versus investigative roles,[47,55] a less research-dominant career pathway. However, these gender differences do not fully explain the differences in research productivity.

Women are more likely to receive significantly less funding than their male counterparts when applying for NIH grants,[56] which may impact their ability to fund projects that would otherwise be submitted for publication. Grant funding also helps attract more trainees, and thus support for research and increased research productivity.[2] Although there is conflicting data on whether women are less successful than men in obtaining grants,[56,57] women frequently receive smaller grants than their male peers,[58,59] which is more pronounced at lower academic ranks.[60] Furthermore, women report having lower institutional support than men,[50] and adequate institutional support of research has been associated with increasing rank for women but not men.[52] Given that research productivity is considered a key measure used in promotional processes,[61,62] this potentially disadvantages otherwise qualified women from being promoted. In turn, this may contribute to the persistence of the dearth of women in leadership positions in academic medicine.[40]

Gender Differences Among Journal Reviewers

Females account for a small percentage of reviewers at peer-reviewed journals. Between 2010 and 2011 females accounted for 25% of the more than 16,000 reviewers across six major medical journals,[63] and almost a decade later account for only 18% of the top 1% most active reviewers, as measured by the number of verified pre-publication reviews completed annually, in the United States.[64] Of top reviewers, women review fewer manuscripts annually, but leave substantially longer reviews than their male counterparts. Given reciprocity preferences in peer review, this might affect the gender representation of authors published in the journal and contribute to persisting gender imbalances.[64] On the other hand, having a female editor-in-chief is associated with not only an increase in the presence of females among the editorial and advisory boards, but also the proportion of females who engage in peer review[65] and the representation of female first authorships[43] emphasizing the downstream effects of gender inequity among leadership positions.

Gender Differences and Journal Editorial Board Composition

Several top dermatology journals have been publishing articles for the past 120 years, but only 19% of the editors-in-chief across these journals have been female.[66] Naomi Kanof was an editor-in-chief at the *Journal of Investigate Dermatology* as early as 1949, however, most journals did not have their first female editor-in-chief until the twenty-first century.[66] As of 2017%, 46% of these journals have had exclusively male editors-in-chief. Of those with at least one female editor-in-chief, only one in five had at least 50% female representation since their first year in publication, including one journal with all female editors-in-chief, the *International Journal of Women's Dermatology* (IJWD).[66]

In 2018, females continued to make up roughly 19% of editors-in-chief across a wide range of dermatology journals,[66] and only 10% of those at top scoring dermatology journals according to SCImago journal rankings.[35] These findings are not unique to dermatology, and the proportion of female editors-in-chief varies greatly across specialties, ranging from 0% to 82%.[65] Overall, the underrepresentation of females as editors-in-chief has remained relatively unchanged since the late 1990s.[67]

There also remains a paucity of women across editorial board positions.[35,44,65,67–70] In 1999, women accounted for less than 19% of editorial board members at top medical journals[67] and constituted only 23% of those in 2011.[68] Seven years later, women continued to account for only 22% of over 5800 editorial board members of dermatology journals with the smallest proportion of women among editors-in-chief (19%) and the highest among deputy editors (42%).[35] This is in stark contrast to the IJWD, which has an editorial board comprised of 83% females, including both editors-in-chief.[42] Likewise, women are more well represented on editorial boards for medical education and women's health journals, where women have occupied approximately 42% of board member positions.[44,69]

The Impact of Gender Norms on Career Advancement

Gender norms can negatively affect the careers of women across many domains. For instance, women with children are more likely to work fewer hours to care for children,[38,53] not necessarily because their goals or aspirations are different from their male peers,[71] but because there are nuanced expectations of men and women that are deeply seeded in society.[2] These expectations can result in gender bias, in which, women shoulder a disproportionate responsibility for childrearing. However, without astutely evaluating the reasons why women with children spend fewer hours at their workplace, it permits a superficial, and seemingly rational, explanation for why women are not represented among academic leadership and are paid less. For example, reduced working hours can result in less time to conduct research and accordingly a decrease in research productivity, a key measure in determining promotions within academic medicine.[61] This evaluation, however, discounts two things: (1) the other factors that contribute to decreased research productivity and (2) the barriers to career advancement women experience that cannot be otherwise explained by the number of hours a physician works.

Women in academic medicine receive less research funding,[72–76] which also plays a significant role in research productivity, by providing physician-researchers with needed funds to support their projects. Although working fewer hours may leave less time to write and submit grant applications, systemic gender-based disadvantages may also play a role in why women receive less funding.[77–79] For instance, a recent study showed that despite male and female university students applying at equal rates for funding to study or conduct research abroad, male students were significantly more likely to be awarded the grant.[79] The study found that when reviewers were blinded to the applicants' genders, there were no significant gender differences in the quality of the applications submitted. These gender-based disadvantages can also be seen in the hiring and promotional processes and can also impact application and performance reviews.[80–82] For instance, one study reported that the inclusion of the word "leader" in tenure criteria was negatively associated with the proportion of tenured women faculty at an institution.[82] Additionally, women may be overlooked by selection committees for promotions based on gender due to a perceived lack of a collegial environment for women as part of a leadership group.[5,81]

Impact of Pregnancy and Parental Leave on Career Advancement

Medical training often coincides with prime childbearing years[83–85]; only 2% of women have their first child before medical school.[84] Unlike men, women have a "biological clock," in which fertility declines with increasing age,[86] creating a delicate balance between biologic needs and the inflexibility of medical training.[87] Although more than half of female dermatologists who choose to have children will have their first child during residency,[84] most women in medicine delay having children by more than 7 years when compared with the general population.[88]

A recent study found that women were significantly less likely to plan on having children during residency than their male counterparts (27% vs 41%, respectively).[89] One in five residents cited concerns over hindering their educational training or career opportunities as reasons for delaying children.[90] Women have also reported concern of the discernment that having children during residency indicates they are less committed to their careers.[84] These perceived consequences are part of the "motherhood penalty," in which mothers face disadvantages in the workplace after having a child based on the false assumption that being a mother and having a successful career are incompatible.[3]

The variability of new parental leave policies across residency training programs and specialties are discussed in detail elsewhere.[83,84,90] Individuals who give birth carry a greater physical postpartum burden and frequently bare more childrearing responsibilities, such as breastfeeding; thus, women who give birth are more likely to experience a greater impact of new parental leave policies as compared with their partners.[83] For some residency programs, this impact includes the potential consequence of having to delay sitting for board exams if a resident misses more than 6 consecutive weeks in a single year.[83] In dermatology, the American Board of Dermatology limits a resident's annual leave to 14 weeks (including vacation time) without considering any complications experienced during pregnancy or the postpartum period.[91] Furthermore, many residents use their elective time, sick time, and/or vacation days to accommodate or extend parental leave.[83,91]

Although many residency programs work with residents to accommodate family planning,[84] the lack of a standardized new parental leave policy generates imbalances that can lead to unfair treatment by preceptors and co-residents.[83] A 10-year study of medicine residents found that female residents who recently gave birth received lower peer evaluation scores than male counterparts who had partners in the postpartum period.[92] This may be secondary to a lack of institutional support leading to an increased workload placed on co-residents while on leave generating animosity,[84] however, these negative effects remain apparent after returning to work, especially for breastfeeding women. In one study, whereas 100% of pregnant residents chose to breastfeed, more than half stopped due to residency obligations.[90] Even if a woman chooses to stop breastfeeding, the pressures of childrearing persist.

Impact of Childrearing and Domestic Responsibilities on Career Advancement

In a study of clinical department chairs, women reported that traditional gender roles, including caring for children, was a major barrier to career advancement.[5] Female physicians with children spend more time childrearing and attending to domestic responsibilities than their male partners,[51,93,94] equating to roughly 8.5 additional hours per week.[51] In fact, male department chairs indicated that the extent of their career success depended on the sacrifices of their partners.[5] Moreover, men's partners contribute significantly more time to tending to domestic tasks compared with women's partners even after adjusting for partner working status.[51] As female physicians are four times more likely than men to have a working partner,[51] this exacerbates the already unequal gender distribution of household responsibilities.

Caring for children is a common key stressor in dual-career households.[4,69] Still, the structure of household responsibilities remains relatively unchanged[4] despite women accounting for roughly half of physicians. Consequently, female physicians are more likely to alter their careers to benefit their families,[95,96] including working less hours.[54] Most women with children who reduce their working hours report that it is secondary to childcare responsibilities.[38,53] One study showed that having children significantly increased the likelihood that women physicians worked part time but made no impact on men's working hours.[54] Other studies have found that male physicians report a significant increase in working hours after having children.[38,97] This may reflect preconceived gender roles, in which women are traditionally expected to raise children and maintain their household,[98] whereas men are to provide financial support by working.[2] Thus, women with children may work less hours compared with men not because they have differing priorities,[3] but rather because of the lack of social support from society needed to address bias stemming from gender roles. This lack of support is not without consequence.

Women must determine how to achieve success in their career in the face of meeting the needs of their families,[95] resulting in an undue burden of managing an asymmetrical division of labor at home while simultaneously taking on the endeavor of climbing the academic ranks.[4,98] One female physician shared that to achieve this, she had to make compromises early in her career, including missing conferences, which could have otherwise served as networking opportunities.[95]

Many women with young children spend less time on research activities, including time spent applying for grant funding and women may focus on publishing full papers instead of abstracts.[69,95] Writing grants and conducting research often require prolonged hours of uninterrupted work that can be difficult to complete if an individual does not have protected time in their schedule for these activities, such as women pursuing less research-dominant career paths. Whereas, conducting other activities in clinical work or mentoring can be short-term and periodic in nature, which may be easier to balance with other responsibilities, including childrearing.

Opportunities for Addressing Gender Inequities in Academic Medicine

Gender inequity spans all domains of academic medicine. Although great strides have been made to identify the disparities that exist, a great deal of work remains to be done. Most, articles cited support this need and several declare a call-to-action.[25,26,77,83,84,99] Given the tightly woven and non-linear relationships between the factors that contribute to persistence of gender inequity in academic medicine, a multifaceted approach is essential to reducing these barriers and for reaching gender parity (Table 2).

Having a mentor early in one's career nearly doubles their chances of being promoted to associate professor within 6 years of becoming an assistant professor for both men and women.[100] Dermatology residency program directors report that mentorship plays a crucial role in a resident's professional development.[101,102] Most mentees find mentorship beneficial, although spontaneous mentorships (ie, mentorship formed through shared interests or positive working relationship) have been reported as more helpful than official mentorships (ie, mentorship formed by assignment) when navigating workplace politics, discussing career progression, and attaining fellowship positions.[101]

Although many women prefer a gender-similar mentor, most mentees indicate that mentors, irrespective of gender, can help with career development.[101] Furthermore, in a study assessing the role of gender on mentor-mentee relationships did not find any significant gender differences in mentee perceptions of mentor support when obtaining a long-term job, navigating workplace politics, or assistance with research publications. However, gender may play a role when navigating more personal matters, including work-life balance and time management.[101]

Thus, although gender may not directly impact the overall success of a mentor-mentee relationship, shared experiences that are more likely to be experienced by a gender-similar mentor may evoke a stronger connection and facilitate more open communication.[101] For instance, a physician who is breastfeeding for the first time may seek advice regarding how to pump during clinic from a mentor who has breastfed previously.

Many strong connections based on similarities can be made with mentors, irrespective of gender,[103–105] and excellent mentorship is often independent of gender.[106] However, men's ability to effectively mentor women may depend on their awareness of barriers that many women may face throughout their careers, such as the impact gender bias has on obtaining leadership roles.[106]

Beyond connectedness, mentees report multiple attributes that help foster a fruitful mentorship, including a mentor's willingness to educate mentees on topics beyond clinical and research domains, such as maintaining work-life balance or navigating workplace politics.[101] To establish a successful mentorship, mentors and mentees should engage in regular meetings,[101,107] set clear expectations in terms of roles and commitments,[87,101,106,108] and willingness of mentors to offer honest, constructive feedback.[101,106] When mentors possess strong skills, such as in communication or negotiation, they can empower mentees to refine these skills themselves and promote career development.[101,106,107]

Mentors should also actively connect their mentees with others in their network to improve visibility and help establish or grow the mentee's professional network, which is often referred to as sponsorship.[101,106] With sponsorship, an influential, and often more senior, person with access to networks and resources in the field (the sponsor) puts forward a protégé and advocates for them on their behalf to improve visibility or to assist with career-advancing opportunities.[109] Therefore, although mentorship often focuses on overall longitudinal personal and professional development, sponsorship is typically episodic and focused on career advancement.[109,110]

There are numerous benefits that can be drawn from having a mentor beyond career advancement, including promoting personal growth and well-being.[88,101,111,112] For women, in particular, this can include having someone to help navigate the challenges that arise throughout pregnancy, raising children, caring for aging parents, or when managing household responsibilities. Having a mentor early in one's career can, in turn, significantly increase the likelihood that a mentee will consider mentoring in the future.[101]

Mentors who connect mentees with others in the field creates an opportunity for mentees to improve their organizational skills as they balance multiple mentorship relationships.[106] Of note, mentorship may help protect mentees from feelings of burnout,[93,113] an important consideration as physicians face high rates of burnout.[114] Formal mentorship programs and organizations (eg, the Women's Dermatology Society's mentorship program) have also sought to raise awareness on gender equality initiatives,[115–117] to help improve gender inequities, such as the underrepresentation of women in leadership by identifying ways to engage women in positive mentoring relationship to support career advancement.[111,117]

Having a positive role model alone can stimulate career-oriented behavior and increase the likelihood of being promoted.[100] The limited number of women in leadership positions within academic medicine results in a dearth of role models and mentors available to guide their younger counterparts on how to combine their career and household obligations. In the absence of a positive role model to identify with, younger women may be left feeling uninspired as they navigate their career and day-to-day responsibilities. Simultaneously, they are left to overcome the barriers of climbing the academic ranks on their own.

The substantial benefits of mentorship will hopefully increase the representation of women as leaders within academic medicine over time and help break the vicious cycle that limits the advancement of women in medicine because they do not have someone in leadership to lean on as role models for mentorship, sponsorship, and career advice.

Given that women are more likely to work fewer hours when raising children early in their career,[38,53,54] more likely to pursue non-research tracks in academic medicine,[47,55] and frequently face gender-based barriers to publishing,[47,56,60] the promotion criteria in academic medicine must be revised. Broader and more inclusive criteria should include measures that reflect leadership ideals beyond research benchmarks, including mentorship (see **Table 2**).[101,115,118]

As men are more likely to have a career sponsor to advocate for them and assist with networking,[106] leadership training may be of particular value to young female faculty,[113,119] and components

Table 2
Constructive solutions for addressing gender inequity in academic medicine

Gender Inequity Addressed		Proposed Solution	Anticipated Impact
Leadership Research Productivity	Underrepresentation of women on editorial and advisory boards → ↓ representation of women in leadership positions and ↓ female authorship	To develop and maintain diversity at all levels of a journal should examine:[42] 1. Author diversity[a] 2. Diversity[a] of editorial and advisory board members 3. How publications support diversity in backgrounds 4. Topics that foster diversity among genders,[b] skin of color, and sexual minority	↑ Diversity of editorial boards → ↑ Women in leadership roles ↑ Diversity of publications → ↑ in female authorship → ↑ in research productivity measures
Pay Gap	↓ starting offers for women and women are less likely to negotiate pay[28,29]	Curricula covering negotiation skills and financial literacy to be incorporated during medical training[28,77] Employers hold accountability to develop rule-based, non-negotiable, standardized salaries[85]	↑ Negotiation skills[113] → Advocate for ↑ pay ↓ Gender-based differences in pay → ↑ Gender equity in pay
Leadership	Promotion criteria emphasize research dominant career tracks → ↓ women mentors in leadership positions	Develop inclusive measures that reflect mentorship as both a form of leadership and productivity[101,115,118]	↑ Promotions among women → ↑ Women in leadership roles ↑ Availability of women mentors in leadership
Childcare Burden	Lack of universal NPL policy → ↑ burden for women to have children in residency and ↓ support from co-residents and faculty in postpartum period	Standardize an NPL policy across residency programs (eg, 8 wk) that is inclusive of support systems for co-residents while resident takes leave[83]	↓ Negative perceptions from co-residents and faculty ↓ Guilt and post-partum burden ↓ Burnout
	Unequal childrearing burden[51] and lack of support[3] → major barrier to career advancement[5,95]	Establishment of hospital-provided, on-site (or near-site) childcare services with extended hours[122]	↑ Childcare support → ↓ Unequal childrearing burden on women → ↓ Impact of childrearing on career[122,123]

[a] Diversity as defined by race, gender, ethnic background, and country of origin.
[b] Including non-binary genders and transgender concerns. NPL: new parental leave.

should include education on conflict resolution,[120] development of strong negotiation skills, and improved ability to navigate politics in the workplace.[101] Leadership training programs may serve as an adjunct to mentorship for young women to help reduce barriers to career advancements.

To reduce the unequal burden of childrearing and household responsibilities women carry, parental leave revisions are needed (see **Table 2**).[83,91,121,122] If programs are not able to sufficiently provide coverage and/or are concerned that a parental leave (eg, 8 week) will significantly impair a resident's ability to be competent at the end of the training, there are much larger concerns about the structure of medical training that need to be addressed.[83]

Established in 2015, the *International Journal of Women's Dermatology* (IJWD) has been extremely successful in maintaining a strong representation of women not only as authors but also as leaders on the editorial board.[42] To address barriers in publishing, the co-editors in chief of the IJWD and co-authors of this paper, Murase and Murrell, offer insights from the perspective of the IJWD (see **Table 2**).[42] These active and proactive efforts promote accountability for journals and academic programs to ensure just representation of men and women across academic medicine. A similar approach can be used to address the gender gap in pay (see **Table 2**).

Many recommendations focus on change at an institutional level. Yet, we can continue spearheading the progression to gender parity in academic medicine as individuals. As Grant-Kels[123] called upon women dermatologists in 2019, we can drive these changes by both running for the American Academy of Dermatology (AAD) board and pursuing leadership positions at places of employment. Petitions can also drive change. In the past, petitioning employers to start an on-campus daycare and petitioning meeting committees to establish daycare programs at conference meetings have been successful. (**Table 2**).

SUMMARY

Since the 1970s, academic dermatology departments have seen improvements in the gender parity of women among more junior positions, such as assistant professor and first authorship in peer-reviewed journals. Fifty years later, there remains a gender gap among more senior academic and leadership positions. Notably, gender parity among dermatology program directors was reached in 2016, indicating that gender gaps among certain leadership roles are improving.

Gender bias continues to contribute to the disproportionate barriers to promotion, equal compensation, and mentorship many women experience in academic medicine, especially when raising children. This contributes to the cyclic process that perpetuates the underrepresentation of women in leadership who could otherwise serve as role models for their younger counterparts. The gender inequity within academic medicine, and dermatology, is a deeply engrained, systemic problem, creating a vicious cycle that will require a multi-faceted approach and commitment from every level of the system to establish and maintain gender equity across positions in academic medicine.

CLINICS CARE POINTS

- Gender inequity spans all domains of academic medicine and will require a multifarious approach for improvement.
- There are key differences in mentorship and sponsorship. While both can have positive implications for one's career, mentorship is often a longitudinal relationship that focuses on both personal and professional development. Conversely, sponsorship is often more directed towards promoting career advancement.
- Many institutions utilize research productivity as a key measure for determining readiness for a promotion. Given that women are less likely to pursue a research dominant career path, promotion criteria should be expanded to be more inclusive of measures that reflect leadership ideals beyond research benchmarks.
- Childrearing has been identified as a major barrier to career advancement for women with children. Multiple approaches, including on-site daycare, standardized new parental leave policies, and reform of promotion criteria have been proposed to help reduce this barrier.
- While many of the proposed recommendations for improving gender equity in academic medicine have been focused on change at an institutional level, individuals can advocate for change by running for leadership positions and creating petitions to address barriers to improving gender equity.

FUNDING

This article has no funding source.

CONFLICT OF INTEREST STATEMENT

None of the authors have any relevant conflicts of interest.

REFERENCES

1. Organization WH. Gender and health. https://www.who.int/health-topics/gender#tab=tab_1. [Accessed 14 March 2022].

2. Tricco AC, Bourgeault I, Moore A, et al. Advancing gender equity in medicine. CMAJ 2021;193(7): E244–50.

3. DeWane ME, Grant-Kels JM. A commentary on gender bias in dermatology and its perceived impact on career development among women dermatologists. Int J Womens Dermatol 2020;6(5):440–4.

4. Rosenthal J, Wanat KA, Samimi S. Striving for balance: A review of female dermatologists' perspective on managing a dual-career household. Int J Womens Dermatol 2020;6(1):43–5.

5. Yedidia MJ, Bickel J. Why aren't there more women leaders in academic medicine? the views of clinical department chairs. Acad Med 2001;76(5):453–65.

6. Feramisco JD, Leitenberger JJ, Redfern SI, et al. A gender gap in the dermatology literature? Cross-sectional analysis of manuscript authorship trends in dermatology journals during 3 decades. J Am Acad Dermatol 2009;60(1):63–9.

7. OCR) OfCR. Title IX of the Education Amendments of 1972. October 27, 2021 October 17, 2019. https://www.hhs.gov/civil-rights/for-individuals/sex-discrimination/title-ix-education-amendments/index.html#:~:text=Title%20IX%20of%20the%20Education%20Amendments%20of%201972%20(Title%20IX,activity%20receiving%20federal%20financial%20assistance. [Accessed 14 March 2022].

8. Schaller JG. The Advancement of Women in Academic Medicine. JAMA 1990;264(14):1854–5.

9. (AAMC) AoAMC. The State of Women in Academic Medicine 2018-2019: Exploring Pathways to Equity. https://store.aamc.org/downloadable/download/sample/sample_id/330/. [Accessed 9 March 2022].

10. Xierali IM, Nivet MA, Pandya AG. US Dermatology Department Faculty Diversity Trends by Sex and Underrepresented-in-Medicine Status, 1970 to 2018. JAMA Dermatol 2020;156(3):280–7.

11. Margosian E. Spotlight on dermatology demographics. Derm World: Navigating Practice, Policy, and Patient Care. Am Acad Dermatol 2022;64.

12. Henderson EF. Sticky care and conference travel: unpacking care as an explanatory factor for gendered academic immobility. Higher Education 2021;82(4):715–30.

13. Lundine J, Bourgeault IL, Clark J, et al. The gendered system of academic publishing. Lancet 2018;391(10132):1754–6.

14. Sadeghpour M, Bernstein I, Ko C, et al. Role of sex in academic dermatology: results from a national survey. Arch Dermatol 2012;148(7):809–14.

15. (AAMC) AoAMC. U.S. Medical School Faculty by Gender, Rank, and Department, 2021. 2021. https://www.aamc.org/media/9736/download?attachment. [Accessed 9 March 2022].

16. (AAMC) AoAMC. Faculty Roster: U.S. Medical School Faculty. https://www.aamc.org/data-reports/faculty-institutions/interactive-data/https/wwwaamcorg/data-reports/faculty-institutions/interactive-data/us-medical-school-deans-trends. [Accessed 7 March 2022].

17. Odei BC, Gawu P, Bae S, et al. Evaluation of Progress Toward Gender Equity Among Departmental Chairs in Academic Medicine. JAMA Intern Med 2021;181(4):548–50.

18. Kuo IC, Levine RB, Gauda EB, et al. Identifying Gender Disparities and Barriers to Measuring the Status of Female Faculty: The Experience of a Large School of Medicine. J Womens Health (Larchmt) 2019;28(11):1569–75.

19. (AAMC) AoAMC. The State of Women in Academic Medicine: Administrative Faculty Leaders by Gender, Rank, and Office. 2018. https://www.aamc.org/sites/default/files/aa-data-reports-state-of-women-administrative-faculty-leaders-rank-office-2018_0.jpg. [Accessed 7 March 2022].

20. Thompson AM, Atluri S, Yee D, et al. Academic dermatology chair and chief characteristics. Int J Womens Dermatol 2021;7(5Part B):860–2.

21. Turner E, Yoo J, Salter S, et al. Leadership workforce in academic dermatology. Arch Dermatol 2007;143(7):948–9.

22. Alikhan A, Ghods M, Armstrong AW. Survey of demographic and educational factors among dermatology chairs and chiefs. Cutis 2012;89(4):195–8.

23. Shi CR, Olbricht S, Vleugels RA, et al. Sex and leadership in academic dermatology: A nationwide survey. J Am Acad Dermatol 2017;77(4):782–4.

24. Kimball AB. Sex, academics, and dermatology leadership: progress made, but no more excuses. Arch Dermatol 2012;148(7):844–6.

25. (AAMC) AoAMC. Gender Equity in Academic Medicine. https://www.aamc.org/news-insights/gender-equity-academic-medicine. [Accessed 7 March 2022].

26. (AAMC) AoAMC. AAMC Statement on Gender Equity. https://www.aamc.org/what-we-do/equity-diversity-inclusion/aamc-statement-gender-equity. [Accessed 7 March 2022].

27. Bowles HR, Babcock L, Lai L. Social incentives for gender differences in the propensity to initiate negotiations: Sometimes it does hurt to ask. Organ Behav Hum Decis Process 2007;103(1):84–103.

28. Catenaccio E, Rochlin JM, Simon HK. Addressing Gender-Based Disparities in Earning Potential in Academic Medicine. JAMA Netw Open 2022;5(2): e220067.

29. Fischer LH, Bajaj AK. Learning How to Ask: Women and Negotiation. Plast Reconstr Surg 2017;139(3): 753–8.

30. Weeks WB, Wallace AE. Gender differences in dermatologists' annual incomes. Cutis 2007;80(4):325–32.

31. Srivastava R, Brancard T, Ashforth GF, et al. Gender Disparities in Income Among Board-Certified Dermatologists. Cutis 2021;108(6):352–6.

32. Sachdeva M, Price KN, Hsiao JL, et al. Gender and rank salary trends among academic dermatologists. Int J Womens Dermatol 2020;6(4):324–6.

33. Jena AB, Olenski AR, Blumenthal DM. Sex Differences in Physician Salary in US Public Medical Schools. JAMA Intern Med 2016;176(9):1294–304.

34. Guss L, Chen Q, Hu C, et al. Income inequality between male and female clinical faculty at public academic dermatology departments. J Am Acad Dermatol 2020;83(2):633–6.

35. Lobl M, Grinnell M, Higgins S, et al. Representation of women as editors in dermatology journals: A comprehensive review. Int J Womens Dermatol 2020;6(1):20–4.

36. Gentle JE. Computational Statistics. In: Peterson P, Baker E, McGaw B, editors. International encyclopedia of education. Third Edition. Oxford: Elsevier; 2010. p. 93–7.

37. Resneck JS Jr, Tierney EP, Kimball AB. Challenges facing academic dermatology: survey data on the faculty workforce. J Am Acad Dermatol 2006; 54(2):211–6.

38. Jacobson CC, Nguyen JC, Kimball AB. Gender and parenting significantly affect work hours of recent dermatology program graduates. Arch Dermatol 2004;140(2):191–6.

39. Laughter MR, Yemc MG, Presley CL, et al. Gender representation in the authorship of dermatology publications. J Am Acad Dermatol 2022;86(3):698–700.

40. Bendels MHK, Dietz MC, Bruggmann D, et al. Gender disparities in high-quality dermatology research: a descriptive bibliometric study on scientific authorships. BMJ Open 2018;8(4):e020089.

41. Ziarati P, Baker C, Dwan D, et al. Representation of women among authors and presenters in contact dermatitis and at the European Society of Contact Dermatitis congresses: A look over 28 years. Contact Dermatitis 2020;83(6):537–8.

42. Murase JE, Murrell DF. Embracing diversity in dermatology: Creation of a culture of inclusion in dermatologic publishing. Int J Womens Dermatol 2021;7(4):371–7.

43. Filardo G, da Graca B, Sass DM, et al. Trends and comparison of female first authorship in high impact medical journals: observational study (1994-2014). BMJ 2016;352:i847.

44. Madden C, O'Malley R, O'Connor P, et al. Gender in authorship and editorship in medical education journals: A bibliometric review. Med Educ 2021;55(6):678–88.

45. Holman L, Stuart-Fox D, Hauser CE. The gender gap in science: How long until women are equally represented? Plos Biol 2018;16(4):e2004956.

46. Broderick NA, Casadevall A. Gender inequalities among authors who contributed equally. Elife 2019;8. https://doi.org/10.7554/eLife.36399.

47. Bendels MHK, Muller R, Brueggmann D, et al. Gender disparities in high-quality research revealed by Nature Index journals. PLoS One 2018; 13(1):e0189136.

48. Shah SGS, Dam R, Milano MJ, et al. Gender parity in scientific authorship in a National Institute for Health Research Biomedical Research Centre: a bibliometric analysis. BMJ Open 2021;11(3):e037935.

49. Larson AR, Poorman JA, Silver JK. Representation of Women Among Physician Authors of Perspective-Type Articles in High-Impact Dermatology Journals. JAMA Dermatol 2019;155(3):386–8.

50. Carr P, Friedman RH, Moskowitz MA, et al. Research, academic rank, and compensation of women and men faculty in academic general internal medicine. J Gen Intern Med 1992;7(4):418–23.

51. Jolly S, Griffith KA, DeCastro R, et al. Gender differences in time spent on parenting and domestic responsibilities by high-achieving young physician-researchers. Ann Intern Med 2014;160(5):344–53.

52. Kaplan SH, Sullivan LM, Dukes KA, et al. Sex differences in academic advancement. Results of a national study of pediatricians. N Engl J Med 1996; 335(17):1282–9.

53. Bansal A, Sarkar R. Women in Dermatology Leadership: Results from a Nationwide Survey. Indian Dermatol Online J 2021;12(6):834–40.

54. Lachish S, Svirko E, Goldacre MJ, et al. Factors associated with less-than-full-time working in medical practice: results of surveys of five cohorts of UK doctors, 10 years after graduation. Hum Resour Health 2016;14(1):62.

55. Wehner MR, Naik HB, Linos E. Gender Equity in Clinical Dermatology-Reason for Optimism. JAMA Dermatol 2019;155(3):284–6.

56. Hechtman LA, Moore NP, Schulkey CE, et al. NIH funding longevity by gender. Proc Natl Acad Sci 2018;115(31):7943–8.

57. Pohlhaus JR, Jiang H, Wagner RM, et al. Sex differences in application, success, and funding rates for NIH extramural programs. Acad Med 2011; 86(6):759–67.

58. Ash AS, Carr PL, Goldstein R, et al. Compensation and advancement of women in academic medicine: is there equity? Ann Intern Med 2004; 141(3):205–12.

59. Rose SL, Sanghani RM, Schmidt C, et al. Gender Differences in Physicians' Financial Ties to Industry: A Study of National Disclosure Data. PLoS One 2015;10(6):e0129197.

60. Waisbren SE, Bowles H, Hasan T, et al. Gender differences in research grant applications and

funding outcomes for medical school faculty. J Womens Health (Larchmt) 2008;17(2):207–14.

61. Jagsi R, Guancial EA, Worobey CC, et al. The "gender gap" in authorship of academic medical literature–a 35-year perspective. N Engl J Med 2006;355(3):281–7.

62. Stossel TP. Volume: papers and academic promotion. Ann Intern Med 1987;106(1):146–9.

63. Erren TC, Groß JV, Shaw DM, et al. Representation of Women as Authors, Reviewers, Editors in Chief, and Editorial Board Members at 6 General Medical Journals in 2010 and 2011. JAMA Intern Med 2014;174(4):633–5.

64. Zhang L, Shang Y, Huang Y, et al. Gender differences among active reviewers: an investigation based on publons. Scientometrics 2022;127(1):145–79.

65. Pinho-Gomes A-C, Vassallo A, Thompson K, et al. Representation of Women Among Editors in Chief of Leading Medical Journals. JAMA Netw Open 2021;4(9). e2123026-e26.

66. Gollins CE, Shipman AR, Murrell DF. A study of the number of female editors-in-chief of dermatology journals. Int J Womens Dermatol 2017;3(4):185–8.

67. Kennedy BL, Lin Y, Dickstein LJ. Women on the editorial boards of major journals. Acad Med 2001;76(8):849–51.

68. Amrein K, Langmann A, Fahrleitner-Pammer A, et al. Women underrepresented on editorial boards of 60 major medical journals. Gend Med 2011;8(6):378–87.

69. Grinnell M, Higgins S, Yost K, et al. The proportion of male and female editors in women's health journals: A critical analysis and review of the sex gap. Int J Womens Dermatol 2020;6(1):7–12.

70. Morton MJ, Sonnad SS. Women on professional society and journal editorial boards. J Natl Med Assoc 2007;99(7):764–71.

71. Grant-Kels JM. Too many female doctors are part-time or stop working. Int J Womens Dermatol 2020; 6(1):37–8.

72. Jagsi R, Motomura AR, Griffith KA, et al. Sex differences in attainment of independent funding by career development awardees. Ann Intern Med 2009; 151(11):804–11.

73. Kaatz A, Lee YG, Potvien A, et al. Analysis of National Institutes of Health R01 Application Critiques, Impact, and Criteria Scores: Does the Sex of the Principal Investigator Make a Difference? Acad Med 2016;91(8):1080–8.

74. Price KN, Collier EK, Atluri S, et al. National Institutes of Health Dermatology Funding Trends 2015-2019. J Invest Dermatol 2021;141(1):232–5.

75. Sege R, Nykiel-Bub L, Selk S. Sex Differences in Institutional Support for Junior Biomedical Researchers. JAMA 2015;314(11):1175–7.

76. Stewart C, Lipner SR. Gender and race trends in academic rank of dermatologists at top U.S. institutions: A cross-sectional study. Int J Womens Dermatol 2020;6(4):283–5.

77. Bates C, Gordon L, Travis E, et al. Striving for Gender Equity in Academic Medicine Careers: A Call to Action. Acad Med 2016;91(8):1050–2.

78. Lewiss RE, Silver JK, Bernstein CA, et al. Is Academic Medicine Making Mid-Career Women Physicians Invisible? J Womens Health (Larchmt) 2020; 29(2):187–92.

79. Wijnen MN, JJM Massen, Kret ME. Gender bias in the allocation of student grants. Scientometrics 2021;126(7):5477–88.

80. Komlenac N, Gustafsson Senden M, Verdonk P, et al. Parenthood does not explain the gender difference in clinical position in academic medicine among Swedish, Dutch and Austrian physicians. Adv Health Sci Educ Theory Pract 2019;24(3): 539–57.

81. Lu JD, Sverdlichenko I, Siddiqi J, et al. Barriers to Diversity and Academic Promotion in Dermatology: Recommendations Moving Forward. Dermatology 2021;237(4):489–92.

82. Marchant A, Bhattacharya A, Carnes M. Can the Language of Tenure Criteria Influence Women's Academic Advancement? J Womens Health (Larchmt) 2007;16(7):998–1003.

83. Ortiz Worthington R, Feld LD, Volerman A. Supporting New Physicians and New Parents: A Call to Create a Standard Parental Leave Policy for Residents. Acad Med 2019;94(11):1654–7.

84. Mattessich S, Shea K, Whitaker-Worth D. Parenting and female dermatologists' perceptions of work-life balance. Int J Women's Dermatol 2017;3(3):127–30.

85. Lester J, Wintroub B, Linos E. Disparities in Academic Dermatology. JAMA Dermatol 2016;152(8): 878–9.

86. Chua SJ, Danhof NA, Mochtar MH, et al. Age-related natural fertility outcomes in women over 35 years: a systematic review and individual participant data meta-analysis. Hum Reprod 2020;35(8): 1808–20.

87. Grant-Kels JM. Mentorship: Opinion of a silver-haired dermatologist. J Am Acad Dermatol 2015; 73(6):1066.

88. Wietsma AC. Barriers to success for female physicians in academic medicine. J Community Hosp Intern Med Perspect 2014;4. https://doi.org/10.3402/jchimp.v4.24665.

89. Willett LL, Wellons MF, Hartig JR, et al. Do Women Residents Delay Childbearing Due to Perceived Career Threats? Acad Med 2010;85(4):640–6.

90. Gracey LE, Cronin M, Shinkai K, et al. Program Director and Resident Perspectives on New Parent Leave in Dermatology Residency. JAMA Dermatol 2018;154(10):1222–5.

91. Peart JM, Klein RS, Pappas-Taffer L, et al. Parental leave in dermatology residency: ethical considerations. J Am Acad Dermatol 2015;73(4): 707–9.

92. Krause ML, Elrashidi MY, Halvorsen AJ, et al. Impact of Pregnancy and Gender on Internal Medicine Resident Evaluations: A Retrospective Cohort Study. J Gen Intern Med 2017;32(6):648–53.

93. Smith J, Abouzaid L, Masuhara J, et al. I may be essential but someone has to look after my kids": women physicians and COVID-19. Can J Public Health 2022;113(1):107–16.

94. Parsons WL, Duke PS, Snow P, et al. Physicians as parents: parenting experiences of physicians in Newfoundland and Labrador. Can Fam Physician 2009;55(8):808–809 e4.

95. Rochon PA, Davidoff F, Levinson W. Women in Academic Medicine Leadership: Has Anything Changed in 25 Years? Acad Med 2016;91(8): 1053–6.

96. Warde C, Allen W, Gelberg L. Physician role conflict and resulting career changes. Gender and generational differences. J Gen Intern Med 1996; 11(12):729–35.

97. Woodward CA, Williams AP, Ferrier B, et al. Time spent on professional activities and unwaged domestic work. Is it different for male and female primary care physicians who have children at home? Can Fam Physician 1996;42:1928–35.

98. Raffi J, Trivedi MK, White L, et al. Work-life balance among female dermatologists. Int J Womens Dermatol 2020;6(1):13–9.

99. Linos E, Wintroub B, Shinkai K. Diversity in the dermatology workforce: 2017 status update. Cutis 2017;100(6):352–3.

100. Beasley BW, Simon SD, Wright SM. A time to be promoted. The Prospective Study of Promotion in Academia (Prospective Study of Promotion in Academia). J Gen Intern Med 2006;21(2):123–9.

101. Lin G, Murase JE, Murrell DF, et al. The impact of gender in mentor-mentee success: Results from the Women's Dermatologic Society Mentorship Survey. Int J Womens Dermatol 2021;7(4):398–402.

102. Donovan JC. A survey of dermatology residency program directors' views on mentorship. Dermatol Online J 2009;15(9):1.

103. Grant-Kels JM. Can men mentor women in the #MeToo era? Int J Womens Dermatol 2018;4(3): 179.

104. Grant-Kels JM. Confessions of a feminist who was mentored by men. Int J Womens Dermatol 2021; 7(4):503–4.

105. Byerley JS. Mentoring in the Era of #MeToo. JAMA 2018;319(12):1199–200.

106. Bickel J. How men can excel as mentors of women. Acad Med 2014;89(8):1100–2.

107. Vassallo A, Walker K, Georgousakis M, et al. Do mentoring programmes influence women's careers in the health and medical research sector? A mixed-methods evaluation of Australia's Franklin Women Mentoring Programme. BMJ Open 2021; 11(10):e052560.

108. Farah RS, Goldfarb N, Tomczik J, et al. Making the most of your mentorship: Viewpoints from a mentor and mentee(,). Int J Womens Dermatol 2020;6(1): 63–7.

109. Ayyala MS, Skarupski K, Bodurtha JN, et al. Mentorship Is Not Enough: Exploring Sponsorship and Its Role in Career Advancement in Academic Medicine. Acad Med 2019;94(1):94–100.

110. Cabrera-Muffly C. Mentorship and Sponsorship in a Diverse Population. Otolaryngol Clin North Am 2021;54(2):449–56.

111. Blattner CM, Johnson K, Young J 3rd. Mentorship in dermatology. J Am Acad Dermatol 2015;73(6): 1067–71.

112. Sambunjak D, Straus SE, Marusic A. Mentoring in academic medicine: a systematic review. JAMA 2006;296(9):1103–15.

113. Yin HL, Gabrilove J, Jackson R, et al. Sustaining the Clinical and Translational Research Workforce: Training and Empowering the Next Generation of Investigators. Acad Med 2015;90(7):861–5.

114. Shanafelt TD, Boone S, Tan L, et al. Burnout and satisfaction with work-life balance among US physicians relative to the general US population. Arch Intern Med 2012;172(18):1377–85.

115. Bergfeld W, Drake L. The Women's Dermatology Society: Physicians, Leaders, Mentors. Int J Womens Dermatol 2015;1(1):2–3.

116. Shannon G, Jansen M, Williams K, et al. Gender equality in science, medicine, and global health: where are we at and why does it matter? Lancet 2019;393(10171):560–9.

117. Vasquez R, Pandya AG. Successful mentoring of women. Int J Womens Dermatol 2020;6(1):61–2.

118. Murrell DF, Ryan TJ, Bergfeld WF. Advancement of women in dermatology. Int J Dermatol 2011;50(5): 593–600.

119. Collins A, Strowd LC. Leading ladies: Why leadership programs are so valuable to female physicians. Int J Women's Dermatol 2020;6(1):54–6.

120. Steen A, Shinkai K. Understanding individual and gender differences in conflict resolution: A critical leadership skill. Int J Women's Dermatol 2020; 6(1):50–3.

121. Reed BR, Callen JP, Freedberg IM, et al. Position paper on family or personal leave, including pregnancy, during residency. J Am Acad Dermatol 2001;45(1):118–9.

122. Snyder RA, Tarpley MJ, Phillips SE, et al. The case for on-site child care in residency training and afterward. J Grad Med Educ 2013;5(3):365–7.

123. Grant-Kels JM. Does gender impact publication opportunities? Int J Womens Dermatol 2019; 5(2):91.

Cultural Competence and Humility

Ramiro Rodriguez, MD[a,b],*, Amit G. Pandya, MD[c,d]

KEYWORDS

- Skin of color • Diversity • Inclusion • Humility • Competence • Cultural

KEY POINTS

- Health disparities adversely affect patients, and with increasing diversity within the United States, they affect an increasingly diverse group of individuals.
- Improving cultural competence and humility are 2 ways dermatologists can help lessen the burden of health care disparities.
- Cultural competence and humility are lifelong processes.
- Joining existing efforts within professional dermatology associations is the first step toward encouraging competence and humility development.

INTRODUCTION

Health disparities are preventable differences in the burden of disease, injury, violence, or opportunities to achieve optimal health as experienced by individuals from underprivileged backgrounds. Complex interactions lead to health disparities; however, they are partially accounted for by the patient-physician relationship.[1] This relationship involves the interplay of cultural, racial, ethnic, and social factors between patients and doctors. Physicians, being at the forefront of health care delivery, must take responsibility to mitigate preventable harm that can arise from patient-physician relationships.

Practicing cultural competence and humility are 2 of the many ways physicians can contribute to reducing disparities among diverse groups of patients. The purpose of this article is to review cultural competence and humility and the positive impact they may bring to patient encounters in dermatology and provide steps for dermatologists to foster competence and humility improvement.

History and Definitions

Cultural competency emerged as a concept during the civil rights movement in the early 1960s. The call to action urged respect and consideration of racial and ethnic inequalities in society.[2] From that time, definitions regarding cultural competence and humility in medicine have varied; however, both have the intention to improve health care delivery and are not mutually exclusive.[3]

Culture, race, and ethnicity are associated terms that require consideration in any discussion of cultural humility. Culture refers to a shared ideological framework among individuals that shapes perception, behavior, and transmission of information between people and their reality. Race concerns thinking of people based on physical characteristics, commonly by shared ancestry. Furthermore, ethnicity encompasses grouping people based on a sociocultural perspective including common history, language, religion, and genealogy.[1]

Within the context of those definitions, improving cultural competence is a process that focuses on knowledge acquisition of a particular

[a] The Department of Internal Medicine, The University of Texas Rio Grande Valley, 1401 E 8th Street, Weslaco, TX 78596, USA; [b] The Department of Dermatology, The University of Colorado Anschutz Medical Campus, Aurora, CO, USA; [c] The Department of Dermatology, Palo Alto Foundation Medical Group, 401 Old San Francisco Road, Sunnyvale, CA 94086, USA; [d] The Department of Dermatology, University of Texas Southwestern Medical Center, 5323 Harry Hines Boulevard, Dallas, TX 75390, USA
* Corresponding author. 1665 Aurora Court 3rd Floor, Room 3232, Aurora, CO 80045.
E-mail address: ramiro.a.rodriguezt@gmail.com

Dermatol Clin 41 (2023) 279–283
https://doi.org/10.1016/j.det.2022.10.004
0733-8635/23/© 2022 Elsevier Inc. All rights reserved.

racial, ethnic, or cultural group; interactional skills; and then developing innovative programs by individuals and systems to provide quality health care to diverse populations.[1] Cultural humility is proposed to be synergistic to competence and describes a lifelong process within individuals encouraging self-evaluation, maintaining an other-oriented interpersonal stance, and addressing inherent power imbalances within interactions.[3] A proposed idea is that cultural competence involves 5 main components (awareness, knowledge, skill, encounters, and desire) and that making an effort to incorporate cultural humility within those components will lead to unconscious application during patient interactions (**Table 1**). The unconscious application of humility would in turn allow physicians to communicate more effectively with diverse groups of patients.

Given the literature available concerning cultural competence, the limitation of using this term must be discussed and reframed. For instance, some scholars consider cultural competence is a finite process that can be achieved.[3] However, if considered through the lens of its 5 components, a person must acknowledge that one cannot be fully culturally aware, knowledgeable, or skilled and will always have new experiences upon which to improve. Thus, cultural competence becomes a lifelong process without an end point when considered with its 5 components and cultural humility.[3]

Clinical Outcomes: Cultural Competence and Humility in the Context of Dermatology

The geographic maldistribution of dermatologists, living conditions predisposing toward adverse disease outcomes, insurance status, and communication barriers between physicians and patients are some of the causes of health disparities in dermatology.[4–6] Within the area of communication, cultural competence and humility are infrequently studied. However, available evidence evaluating race and ethnicity concordance within dermatology provides a view of how competence and humility influence clinical outcomes.

In a cross-sectional review of patient encounters evaluating concordance of race, gender, and primary medication nonadherence, Black patients were 11% more likely to receive their medications after seeing a Black provider when compared with non-Black providers (95% confidence interval, -0.2, -0.01).[7] Another cross-sectional survey study was performed with Black patients in focus groups to discuss their experiences in receiving care in a skin of color clinic

and compare those with previous experiences in non–skin of color clinics. Patients reported higher levels of satisfaction, perceived greater respect and dignity, and had increased trustworthiness with their provider after visiting a skin of color clinic. The themes that were highlighted regarding the provider by patients were positive interaction style, perceived fund of knowledge of black skin and hair, and an increased sense of partnership.[8] These findings are similar to previous work that showed lower levels of perceived patient decision making within nonconcordant patient-physician interactions.[9]

Differences involving language also affect patients within dermatology. For instance, in a prospective review of pediatric teledermatology visits, Spanish-speaking patients had significantly fewer scheduled appointments (9% vs 5%, $P<.001$), were less likely to have an e-mail address documented within the electronic medical record (45% vs 62%, $P = .017$), and were less likely to activate their online patient portal (23% vs 66%, $P < .001$).[10] These findings in teledermatology are particularly problematic in patients with diseases requiring early intervention, such as melanoma. One study on racial disparities in melanoma showed that although all minority groups are disproportionately affected, Latinx patients were the only group that experienced a worsening disparity across all disease stages.[11]

Although patient-physician racial/ethnic concordance is important, it is only one factor among many that influence patient encounters.[12] A positive emotional affect, using an open body position, and smile and touch gestures are characteristics of encounters that positively enhance racial-/ethnic-concordant and -discordant interactions.[9] Identifying the manner in which to apply these communication strategies among different ethnic, cultural, and racial groups of patients is an important part of developing better cultural competence and humility.[13]

Future Directions and Conclusion: Fostering Cultural Competence and Humility

Fostering an environment of cultural humility requires opportunities to practice the components of cultural competence. Several recent efforts have been made to facilitate this goal.[14] Multiple dermatology organizations, including the American Academy of Dermatology (AAD), Association of Professors of Dermatology, Society for Investigative Dermatology, Skin of Color Society, Women's Dermatologic Society, American Society of Dermatologic Surgery, Society for Pediatric

Table 1
Culture and medicine definitions

Cultural competence	A process made up of 5 components emphasizing knowledge acquisition of oneself, a particular race, ethnicity, and cultural group, and interactional skills development within those groups
Cultural humility	A process within individuals focused on self-evaluation, maintaining an other-oriented interpersonal stance, and addressing inherent power imbalances within interactions
Cultural awareness	Process of self-reflection and acknowledging one's own biases, upbringing, and how those contrast with others' experiences
Cultural knowledge	Process of obtaining an educational base about beliefs, values, and practices regarding health, incidence and prevalence of disease, and treatment efficacy among diverse groups
Cultural skill	An ability to create a safe environment, ask questions, and seek feedback to gain insight into other cultures in a culturally sensitive manner
Cultural encounters	Interactions with patients from culturally diverse backgrounds during which health care providers are open to encounters as an opportunity for inquisitiveness, self-reflection, critique, and lifelong learning
Cultural desire	The motivation and drive toward improving health care inequities that comes from acknowledging the conditions afflicting underprivileged individuals from different cultures

Dermatology, American Contact Dermatitis Society, and the American Society of Dermatopathology, have developed programs to cultivate cultural awareness, knowledge, skill, and increase diversity within dermatology.

Diversity in medicine is a complex subject that affects many areas of health care. Within the context of fostering cultural competence and humility, increasing diversity within residency programs provides an opportunity for residents to practice the components of cultural competence with their peers. A culturally diversified group of residents can improve the cultural education of all residents through increased cultural interactions with one another. To increase diversity, the AAD published key action items. These action items focus on increasing representation at the medical school level, fostering an interest in dermatology among medical students, and increasing the number of underrepresented in medicine residents in dermatology residency programs.[14] The Skin of Color Society has implemented interventions targeting the pillars of education, research, and mentorship that address these action items. Among the efforts are scientific annual symposia, mentorship opportunities, research grants, and educational curricula to address inadequate training for skin conditions important to individuals with skin of color. These efforts are echoed by the aforementioned organizations and are broadening to include members of the Lesbian, Gay, Bisexual, Transexual, Queer, Intersexual, and asexual (LGBTQIA+) community.[15] More information regarding the AAD key action items, diversity efforts, and the Skin of Color Curriculum can be found at www.aad.org/member/career/diversity.

Participation in these efforts is crucial and forms a starting point toward addressing health disparities. By extension, the future of fostering cultural competence and humility is the application of what is learned in those experiences. Among ways that dermatologists can work toward applying awareness, knowledge, and skill is to expand skin of color clinics. Since the establishment of the first Skin of Color Clinic in 1999, these centers have provided specialized culturally sensitive care for Black, Latinx, and Asian patients; furthered the understanding of the conditions affecting them; and educated many trainees.[12] There are now 15 centers within the United States; however, these will be unlikely to meet the need of the projected minority-majority of Americans by 2044.[16,17]

Despite the challenges ahead, dermatology is among the leading specialties working toward change.[18] The admirable efforts built through decades would have not been possible without people exhibiting the most important characteristic of cultural competence: cultural desire. Incorporating cultural desire is to understand and be committed to addressing inequities in health care. This characteristic is founded on the development of cultural awareness, knowledge, skill, and seeking cultural encounters; it is the drive for dermatologists to "want to" as opposed to "have to."[3] The drive is often associated with a passion for equity and inclusion as a result of acknowledging the unjust conditions afflicting our patients. Dermatologists can lead the way by coming together, understanding social determinants of health that affect our patients, and continuing to strive toward serving all patients, regardless of race or ethnicity, with equality.[12]

SUMMARY

Health disparities disproportionately affect individuals from underprivileged backgrounds who have an array of different cultures. Improving cultural competence and cultural humility are 2 ways in which dermatologists help lessen the burden of health disparities for patients. Fostering cultural awareness, knowledge, and skills through organizations may serve as a starting point. Aims toward augmenting diversity within dermatology and increasing skin of color clinics can provide opportunities for competence and humility development. In turn, the development of better cultural competence and humility will improve understanding of health care disparities and promote a commitment to addressing inequities in health care.

CLINICS CARE POINTS

- Differences in health care delivery can be influenced by patient-physician racial-/ethnic- concordance
- Diversity within residency training programs can help residents improve cultural competence and humility
- Seeking opportunities to improve cultural competence and humility through professional organizations is an important step towards understanding health disparities

FUNDING

The authors did not receive financial support for the research, authorship, and/or publication of this article. Dr. Rodriguez is a post-doctoral fellow at The University of Colorado Anschutz Medical Campus who is funded by the NIH (Grant Number: T32AR007411-37) and an editoral board member for The Journal of Medical Internet Research (JDerm).

DISCLOSURE

The authors do not have any conflicts of interest to disclose.

REFERENCES

1. McKesey J, Berger TG, Lim HW, et al. Cultural competence for the 21st century dermatologist practicing in the United States. J Am Acad Dermatol 2017;77(6):1159–69.
2. Ingleby D, Chiarenza A. Developments in the concept of 'cultural competence. In: Chiarenza A, Devillé W, Kotsioni I, editors. Inequalities in health care for migrants and ethnic minorities. Antwerpen (Apeldoorn): Garant; 2012. p. 66–81.
3. Campinha-Bacote J. Cultural competemility: a paradigm shift in the cultural competence versus cultural humility debate – part I. OJIN: Online J Issues Nurs 2018;24(1). https://doi.org/10.3912/ojin.vol24no01p pt20.
4. Feng H, Berk-Krauss J, Feng PW, et al. Comparison of dermatologist density between urban and rural counties in the United States. JAMA Dermatol 2018;154(11):1265–71.
5. Bray JK, Cline A, McMichael AJ, et al. Differences in healthcare barriers based on racial and/or ethnic background for patients with psoriasis. J Dermatolog Treat 2021;32(6):590–4.
6. Tackett KJ, Jenkins F, Morrell DS, et al. Structural racism and its influence on the severity of atopic dermatitis in African American children. Pediatr Dermatol 2020;37(1):142–6.
7. Adamson AS, Glass DA 2nd, Suarez EA. Patient-provider race and sex concordance and the risk for medication primary nonadherence. J Am Acad Dermatol 2017;76(6):1193–5.
8. Gorbatenko-Roth K, Prose N, Kundu RV, et al. Assessment of Black Patients' perception of their dermatology care. JAMA Dermatol 2019;155(10):1129.
9. Harvey VM, Ozoemena U, Paul J, et al. Patient-provider communication, concordance, and ratings of care in dermatology: Results of a cross-sectional study. Dermatol Online J 2016;22(11). 13030/qt06j6p7gh.

10. Blundell AR, Kroshinsky D, Hawryluk EB, et al. Disparities in telemedicine access for Spanish-speaking patients during the COVID-19 crisis. Pediatr Dermatol 2021;38(4):947–9.

11. Qian Y, Johannet P, Sawyers A, et al. The ongoing racial disparities in melanoma: An analysis of the surveillance, epidemiology, and end results database (1975-2016). J Am Acad Dermatol 2021; 84(6):1585–93.

12. Taylor SC. Meeting the unique dermatologic needs of black patients. JAMA Dermatol 2019;155(10): 1109–10.

13. Grayson C, Heath C. An approach to examining tightly coiled hair among patients with hair loss in race-discordant patient-physician interactions. JAMA Dermatol 2021;157(5):505–6.

14. Pritchett EN, Pandya AG, Ferguson NN, et al. Diversity in dermatology: Roadmap for improvement. J Am Acad Dermatol 2018;79(2):337–41.

15. Desai SR, Khanna R, Glass D, et al. Embracing diversity in dermatology: Creation of a culture of equity and inclusion in dermatology. Int J Women's Dermatol 2021;7(4):378–82.

16. Colby SL, Ortman JM. Projections of the size and composition of the U.S. population: 2014 to 2060. Current Population Reports P25-1143. Washington, DC: U.S. Census Bureau; 2014.

17. Tull RZ, Kerby E, Subash JJ, et al. Ethnic skin centers in the United States: Where are we in 2020? J Am Acad Dermatol 2020;83(6):1757–9.

18. Bray JK, McMichael AJ, Huang WW, et al. Publication rates on the topic of racial and ethnic diversity in dermatology versus other specialties. Dermatol Online J 2020;26(3). 13030/qt094243gp.

Unconscious Bias

Temitayo A. Ogunleye, MD, MHCI

KEYWORDS

- Unconscious bias • Implicit bias • Dermatology • Diversity

KEY POINTS

- Unconscious bias is ubiquitous and affects everyone.
- Implicit bias in health care can reduce the diversity of the field, contribute to professional inequities, and worsen health disparities.
- Intentional effort and programming are necessary to recognize and overcome unconscious bias.

DEFINITIONS (PARTIALLY DERIVED FROM HTTPS://PERCEPTION.ORG/RESEARCH)

Blinding is the removal of all identifiable potentially bias-inducing information, such as race, gender, name, and so forth.

Counter-stereotypic imaging is imagining the individual as the opposite of the stereotype.

Discretion elimination is used when decisions that would normally be made with discretion are instead made using objective criteria.

Explicit bias is an attitude or belief about a person or group on a conscious level.

Identity differences are aspects of people, such as race, ethnicity, gender, sexual orientation, religion, ability, or class, that result in sorting ourselves and others into groups.

Implicit Association Test is a computer-based system to measure automatic associations between concepts. Project Implicit (https://implicit.harvard.edu/implicit/takeatest.html) provides tools to assess a variety of biases, including race, sex, weight, and sexual orientation.

Implicit bias (also called unconscious bias) is a reflexive association of stereotypes or attitudes about groups, often without conscious awareness.

Individuation is seeing the person as an individual rather than a stereotype.

Microaggressions are statements, actions, or incidents with indirect or subtle discrimination against members of a marginalized group.

Stereotype threat occurs when a person is concerned that they will confirm a negative stereotype about their group.

BACKGROUND

The overall racial and ethnic diversity of the United States is shifting. According to the 2020 census data, population growth has mostly slowed in the last decade, but growth that occurred was composed entirely of black, Latino, Asian, and multiracial populations, with white populations declining for the first time on record.[1] It has been projected that by 2050, the United States will become a "majority minority," with minority groups collectively outnumbering white populations.[2] Currently, US census data estimate that that the prevalence of white, African American, Latino, and American Indian/Native American individuals in the US population is 60%, 13.4%, 18.5%, and 1.3%, respectively.[3] There are also notable demographic shifts in sexual orientation and gender identification, with those identifying as a sexual and gender minority doubling from 3.5% to 7.8% in the last 10 years.[4] Nearly 1 in 5 of Generation Z (individuals born between 1997 and 2012) adults identify as lesbian/gay/bisexual/transgender/queer (LGBTQ) according to recent Gallup polls.[4]

MEDICAL WORKFORCE

This shift in diversity has not been accompanied by a correspondent increase in diversity in some medical specialties. "Underrepresented in Medicine," as defined by the Association of American Medical Colleges (AAMC), are those racial and ethnic populations that are underrepresented in the medical profession relative to their numbers

Perelman School of Medicine at the University of Pennsylvania, 3737 Market Street, 11th Floor, Philadelphia, PA 19104, USA
E-mail address: Temitayo.ogunleye@pennmedicine.upenn.edu

Dermatol Clin 41 (2023) 285–290
https://doi.org/10.1016/j.det.2022.08.003

in the general population."[5] According to physician data from the AAMC, 56.2% identified as white, 17.1% identified as Asian, 5.8% identified as Hispanic, 5.0% identified as black or African American, 0.3% identified as American Indian/Native American, and 0.1% identified as Pacific Islander.[6] In 2018, 64.1% of physicians were men, and only 35.8% were women, and specifically in academics, medical school faculty continued to be predominantly white (63.9%) and male (58.6%), especially at the professor and associate professor ranks.[6] The AAMC does not provide data on LGBTQ demographics in the physician workforce.

Dermatology is among the least ethnically/racially diverse specialties despite efforts to improve these demographics. Only 4.2% of dermatologists are Hispanic and 3% of dermatologists are black, far below the national demographics.[7] White dermatologists represent 67.9% of the academic dermatology workforce, and 78.7% and 79.2% represent chair and full professor positions, respectively.[8]

Diversification of the health care workforce is encouraged to help reduce health disparities, particularly those that may be due to unconscious bias.

UNCONSCIOUS/IMPLICIT BIAS

Unconscious biases (also known as implicit biases) are involuntary stereotypes or attitudes held about certain groups of people that may influence our behaviors, understandings, and actions, often with unintended detrimental consequences. The term was initially introduced by psychologists Mahzarin Banaji and Anthony Greenwald,[9] who proposed that social behavior is heavily influenced by unconscious associations and judgments. Implicit bias is ubiquitous and may be incompatible with a person's conscious values or beliefs. Evolutionarily, this reflexive identification of identity differences may have had some survival benefit to allow people to identify potential dangers.[10] However, in current times, explicit and implicit bias within health care can lead to disparities that have real consequences in medical school admissions and education, patient care, faculty hiring, and promotion.[11,12]

MEDICAL SCHOOL ADMISSIONS AND EDUCATION

Implicit bias appears in multiple facets of the education and training of our medical students and trainees, including the application process.

Letters of reference (LOR) play an important role in the ability for medical students or residency applicants to be chosen for their respective programs. One study found evidence of gender bias after analyzing 460 letters of recommendation for urology residency. "Letters for male applicants (were) written in a more authentic tone compared to letters written for female applicants...and contained significantly more references to personal drive, work, and power than letters written for female applicants...Letters of recommendation written about men contained more words referencing drive, work, and power; words typically associated with leadership and professionalism."[13] Another study looking at race-based bias found that traditional letters for non-white applicants had significantly more "grindstone adjectives" highlighting effort (eg, diligent, dedicated, hardworking, persistent) and significantly fewer "standout" adjectives highlighting achievement (eg, superb, amazing, outstanding, remarkable).[14]

Even the process of evaluating the clinical performance of students/trainees can be fraught with bias. Honor society memberships, such as Alpha Omega Alpha (AΩA), have been found to favor white students, with 1 study finding that the odds of AΩA membership for white medical students were nearly 6 times greater than those for black medical students and nearly 2 times greater than for Asian medical students.[15] These findings have led to elimination of several AOA chapters and improvement of the AΩA nomination processes at some medical schools.

Gender and racial/ethnic differences in descriptors in the Medical Student Performance Evaluations (MSPE) have also been described. A study of 6000 US student MSPEs found that white applicants were more likely to be described with "outstanding," "exceptional," and "best" when compared with blacks, Asians, and Hispanics. Similar to findings in LOR gender-based bias, women were more likely to be described with words such as "kind," "caring," and "empathic."[16] One school that examined their clerkship grading schema found that "Black students were less likely to receive honors as compared with White medical students in all 6 clinical core clerkships."[17] These subtle inequities in LORs and clerkship grading can significantly influence the applicant's success in matching for residency, reducing efforts to diversify the workforce.

PATIENT/PROVIDER INTERACTIONS

Implicit bias can have negative effects on provider communication, which can affect patients' trust and satisfaction in their medical care and potentially affect the quality of the health care delivered. Medical education encourages providers to begin clinical presentations of patients with descriptors such as race, age, gender, and sexual identity, which may trigger implicit bias and have implications for care. These reflexive learning associations, such as the "40-year-old black woman with sarcoidosis," or the "darker skinned patient with chancre diagnosed with syphilis," may cause providers to narrow their differential diagnoses and limit treatment options for patients. Although it has been argued that skin color/ethnicity/religion may be important in determining appropriate treatment (eg, darker-skinned patients who may develop hypopigmentation after cryotherapy or a Muslim or Orthodox Jewish woman who may prefer a female provider),[18] assumptions regarding propriety of care based on these identities may still encourage improper care. Using Fitzpatrick Skin Type (FST) may also trigger implicit bias when providers conflate race and ethnicity with FST.[19] Although these learning associations "may be based on true prevalence rates, (they) may not apply to individual patients. Using stereotypes in this fashion may lead to premature closure and missed diagnoses, when clinicians fail to see their patients as more than their perceived demographic characteristics."[20]

This bias may also be seen in medical documentation. Using stigmatizing language, such as "frequent flyer" or "difficult patient," can influence care and outcomes.[21,22] One study examining the effects of stigmatizing language on care provided by medical students and residents used a "randomized vignette study of two chart notes employing stigmatizing versus neutral language to describe the same hypothetical patient."[22] "Exposure to the stigmatizing language note was associated with more negative attitudes toward the patient...and less aggressive management of the patient's pain."[22]

Sun and colleagues[23] analyzed electronic health records (EHRs) for potentially stigmatizing language in the EHRs and its association with race and ethnicity.[23] Analysis of nearly 40,000 hospital notes revealed that black people were 2.54 times more likely to have a negative descriptor in their note. Other groups that were found to have negatively stigmatizing descriptors were patients with Medicaid or Medicare (compared with patients with private or employer-based insurance) and unmarried patients (compared with married patients).[23] These findings remained even after controlling for sociodemographic and health characteristics.

PATIENT SATISFACTION

It has been suggested that race/gender dyad (provider/patient) concordance may lead to better health outcomes, reduced disparities, and improved patient satisfaction. Literature suggests that black patients may experience poorer communication with their providers, some which may be rooted in lack of familiarity with their cultural skin or hair care practices and failure of dermatologists to offer individualized treatments for their disorders.[24,25] Stereotype threat is another component that has the potential to influence patient satisfaction. Stereotype threat refers to the risk of confirming negative stereotypes about an individual's group and may be triggered by microaggressions, defined as a "subtle comment or action that ...unconsciously or unintentionally expresses implicit bias toward a member of a marginalized group."[25] Stereotype threat may be evoked only by patient/provider discordance, leading to "avoidance, disengagement, and distrust that affects follow through with provider recommendations."[24] The Press Ganey (PG) Outpatient Medical Practice Survey is used by many practices as a measure of patient satisfaction, and a cross-sectional analysis of PG surveys from outpatient visits within the University of Pennsylvania Health System between 2014 and 2017 was performed to evaluate the effect on patient/provider concordance on patient satisfaction scores.[26] Racial/ethnic discordance was associated with a lower likelihood of physicians receiving a maximum score, and black and Asian race were both associated with lower patient experience ratings. Gender discordance did not affect PG scoring.[27]

IMPLICIT RACIAL/ETHNIC BIAS AND DERMATOLOGIC-SPECIFIC HEALTH DISPARITIES AND OUTCOMES

Notable health disparities exist among minority groups in the United States, which may be partly attributable to implicit bias. This bias may affect patient/provider communication and satisfaction, but more importantly, may influence patient outcomes and treatment recommendations. One recent cohort study of nearly 30,000 patients examined the effect of race/ethnicity and gender on prescribing patterns for acne.[28] Black patients were less likely than white patients to receive systemic treatments, such as oral antibiotics, hormonal therapy, or isotretinoin, despite being more likely to see a dermatologist.[28] Similar treatment patterns were seen for Asian and Hispanic patients, who were less likely than white patients to receive oral antibiotics/oral contraceptives and oral contraceptives, respectively.[28] These disparities persisted even when controlling for sociodemographic factors, such as mean household income. Given that there are no studies that support difference in racial/ethnic acne severity,[29] the investigators posit that other factors, such as risk aversion,[30,31] medical distrust,[32,33] and physician bias[34] (implicit or explicit), may be affecting treatment recommendations.

Similar discrepancies exist in the treatment of melanoma. Although patients in minority groups have an overall lower incidences of skin cancer, patients from black, Latino, and Asian populations may have higher levels of morbidity and mortality. Specifically, delayed time from diagnosis to definitive surgery is associated with increased melanoma-specific mortality.[35] Bourdeaux and colleagues found that even when sociodemographic factors, including insurance type, were controlled for, black patients were twice as likely to wait 41 to 60 days for treatment, 3 times as likely to wait for 61 to 90 days, and 5 times more likely to wait more than 90 days for definitive surgery.[35] Factors such as differences in disease characteristics (eg, controversies in the care of acral lentiginous melanomas)[35] may partly explain such disparities, but implicit bias are likely an underlying contributing factor.

INTERVENTIONS

There have been many interventions designed to reduce unconscious bias, but few have evidence to support them. Diversity/implicit bias training programs are widely available in many organizations, including hospitals, universities, medical schools, and various corporations. Most of these training programs have a 2-pronged approach of first providing education in the form of defining implicit bias and describing its detrimental effects with the goal of reducing this bias.[36] However, basic social psychology research suggests that education and increased awareness alone do not result in reductions of unconscious bias.[37]

The second component of this approach is to explicitly reduce implicit bias through methods such as deliberate thinking, counter-stereotypic effect, individuation, or meditating before decision making, but there is lacking evidence that these strategies work.[36] Furthermore, there is no evidence that these methods improve the overall goal of improving the quality of care of patients from stigmatized groups.[38] Most programs evaluate effectiveness by survey assessments or retaking the Implicit Association Test, but a 2019 meta-analysis suggests that improvement in scores does not equate to changes in behaviors.[39]

Two strategies that do not require a "conscious override" of unconscious discriminatory behaviors include blinding and discretion elimination. Blinding can be an effective strategy to reduce bias

based on demographic characteristics.[40] Discretion elimination is used when decisions that would normally be made with discretion are instead made using "predetermined, objective criteria that are rigorously applied."[36] "Discretion can be sharply reduced when decision makers precommit to valid decision criteria before they conduct evaluations."[41]

SUMMARY

Implicit bias is ubiquitous and can affect every facet of health care, ultimately impacting the quality of care provided to patients. The reduction of unconscious bias, although difficult, is necessary to improve equity in the field and improve health disparities. Although there is little evidence supporting the effectiveness of current bias/diversity training programming, standardization and blinding may be helpful, evidence-based methods to reduce implicit bias.

DISCLOSURE

No relevant conflicts of interest. T.A. Ogunleye: Janssen Pharmaceuticals Advisory Board.

REFERENCES

1. Tavernise Sabrina, Gebeloff Robert. Census Shows Sharply Growing Numbers of Hispanic, Asian and Multiracial Americans." The New York Times, The New York Times. 2021. Available at: www.nytimes.com/2021/08/12/us/us-census-population-growth-diversity.html. Accessed April 1, 2022.
2. Minorities expected to be majority in 2050. Available at: https://www.cnn.com/2008/US/08/13/census.minorities/. Accessed April 1, 2022.
3. U.S. Census Bureau quickFacts: United States. https://www.census.gov/quickfacts/fact/table/US/PST045221. Accessed May 2, 2022.
4. Jones JM. LGBT identification in U.S. ticks up to 7.1%. Gallup.com. 2022. Available at: https://news.gallup.com/poll/389792/lgbt-identification-ticks-up.aspx. Accessed May 2, 2022.
5. Association of American Medical Colleges. Underrepresented in medicine definition. Available at: https://www.aamc.org/initiatives/urm/. Accessed 10 April 2022.
6. Association of American Medical Colleges (AAMC). AAMC facts & figures 2019; diversity in medical education. Available at: http://www.aamcdiversityfactsandfigures2019.org/index.html. Accessed 10 April 2022.
7. Pandya AG, Alexis AF, Berger TG, et al. Increasing racial and ethnic diversity in dermatology: A call to action. J Am Acad Dermatol 2016;74(3):584–7.

8. Lu JD, Tiwana S, Das P, et al. Gender and racial underrepresentation in academic dermatology positions in the United States: A retrospective, cross sectional study from 2007 to 2018. J Am Acad Dermatol 2020;83(5):1513–6.

9. Banaji MR, Greenwald AG. Implicit gender stereotyping in judgments of fame. J Pers Soc Psychol 1995;68(2):181.

10. Banaji MR, Greenwald AG. Blindspot: hidden biases of good people. 1st edition. USA: Delacorte Press; 2013.

11. Byington CL, Lee V. Addressing disparities in academic medicine: Moving forward. JAMA 2015;314: 1139–41.

12. Smedley BD, Stith Butler A, Bristow LR. In the nation's compelling interest: ensuring diversity in the health-care workforce. Washington, DC: National Academies Press; 2004.

13. Filippou P, Mahajan S, Deal A, et al. The Presence of Gender Bias in Letters of Recommendations Written for Urology Residency Applicants. Urology 2019; 134:56–61. https://doi.org/10.1016/j.urology.2019. 05.065.

14. Powers A, Gerull KM, Rothman R, et al. Race- and Gender-Based Differences in Descriptions of Applicants in the Letters of Recommendation for Orthopaedic Surgery Residency. JB JS Open Access 2020;5(3). e20.00023.

15. Boatright D, Ross D, O'Connor P, et al. Racial Disparities in Medical Student Membership in the Alpha Omega Alpha Honor Society. JAMA Intern Med 2017;177(5):659–65.

16. Ross DA, Boatright D, Nunez-Smith M, et al. Differences in words used to describe racial and gender groups in Medical Student Performance Evaluations. PLoS One 2017;12(8):e0181659.

17. Colson ER, Pérez MA, Blaylock L, et al. Washington University School of Medicine in St. Louis Case Study: A Process for Understanding and Addressing Bias in Clerkship Grading. Acad Med 2020; 95(12S):S131–5.

18. Farshchian M, Grant-Kels JM. Ethics of documenting patient's race and ethnicity in dermatology clinical notes and presentations. J Am Acad Dermatol 2022. S0190-9622(22)00274-282.

19. Ware OR, Dawson JE, Shinohara MM, et al. Racial limitations of Fitzpatrick skin type. Cutis 2020; 105(2):77–80.

20. Jasmine RM, Dawd SS, Victor Robert, et al. The Impact of Unconscious Bias in Healthcare: How to Recognize and Mitigate It. J Infect Dis 2019; 220(Supplement_2). S62–S73.

21. Carroll S. Respecting and empowering vulnerable populations: contemporary terminology. J Nurse Pract 2019;15(3):228–31.

22. Goddu PA, O'Conor KJ, et al. Do Words Matter? Stigmatizing Language and the Transmission of Bias in the Medical Record. J Gen Intern med 2018;33:685–91.

23. Sun M, Oliwa T, Peek ME, et al. Negative Patient Descriptors: Documenting Racial Bias In The Electronic Health Record. Health Aff (Millwood) 2022;41(2): 203–11.

24. Taylor SC. Meeting the Unique Dermatologic Needs of Black Patients. JAMA Dermatol 2019;155(10): 1109–10.

25. Shen MJ, Peterson EB, Costas-Muñiz R, et al. The effects of race and racial concordance on patient–physician communication: A systematic review of the literature. J Racial Ethn Health Disparities 2018;5(1):117–40.

26. Wilson BN, Murase J, Slikwa D, et al. Bridging racial differences in the clinical encounter: How implicit bias and stereotype threat contribute to health care disparities in the dermatology clinic. Int J women's Dermatol 2021;7:2 139–144.

27. Takeshita J, Wang S, Loren AW, et al. Association of Racial/Ethnic and Gender Concordance Between Patients and Physicians With Patient Experience Ratings. JAMA Netw Open 2020;3(11). e2024583.

28. Barbieri JS, Shin DB, Wang S, et al. Association of Race/Ethnicity and Sex With Differences in Health Care Use and Treatment for Acne. JAMA Dermatol 2020;156(3):312–9.

29. Callender VD, Alexis AF, Daniels SR, et al. Racial differences in clinical characteristics, perceptions and behaviors, and psychosocial impact of adult female acne. J Clin Aesthet Dermatol 2014;7(7):19–31.

30. Gorelick J, Daniels SR, Kawata AK, et al. Acne-related quality of life among female adults of different races/ethnicities. J Dermatol Nurses Assoc 2015;7(3):154–62.

31. Constantinescu F, Goucher S, Weinstein A, et al. Understanding why rheumatoid arthritis patient treatment preferences differ by race. Arthritis Rheum 2009;61(4):413–8.

32. Boulware LE, Cooper LA, Ratner LE, et al. Race and trust in the health care system. Public Health Rep 2003;118(4):358–65. https://doi.org/10.1016/S0033-3549(04)50262-5.

33. LaVeist TA, Nickerson KJ, Bowie JV. Attitudes about racism, medical mistrust, and satisfaction with care among African American and white cardiac patients. Med Care Res Rev 2000;57(suppl 1):146–61.

34. Hall WJ, Chapman MV, Lee KM, et al. Implicit racial/ethnic bias among health care professionals and its influence on health care outcomes: a systematic review. Am J Public Health 2015;105(12):e60–76.

35. Tripathi R, Archibald LK, Mazmudar RS, et al. Racial differences in time to treatment for melanoma. J Am Acad Dermatol 2020;83(3):854–9.

36. Greenwald AG, Lai CK. Implicit Social Cognition. Annu Rev Psychol 2020;71:419–45. https://doi.org/10.1146/annurev-psych-010419-050837.

37. Fiske ST. The continuum model and the stereotype content mode. In: Van Lange PAM, Kruglanski AW, Higgins ET, editors. Handbook of theories of social psychologyvol. 1. Sage Publications; 2012. p. 267–88.

38. Hagiwara N, Kron FW, Scerbo MW, et al. A call for grounding implicit bias training in clinical and translational frameworks. Lancet 2020;395(10234): 1457–60.

39. Forscher PS, Lai CK, Axt JR, et al. A meta-analysis of procedures to change implicit measures. J Pers Soc Psychol 2019;117:522–59.

40. Goldin C, Rouse C. Orchestrating impartiality: the impact of "blind" auditions on female musicians. Am Econ Rev 2000;90:715–41.

41. Uhlmann EL, Cohen GL. Constructed criteria: redefining merit to justify discrimination. Psychol Sci 2015;16:474–80.

Understanding and Addressing Microaggressions in Medicine

Michelle Weir, MD

KEYWORDS

- Microaggression • Provider–patient communication • Communication skills
- Addressing microaggressions

KEY POINTS

- Microaggressions are delivered unconsciously either through words, tone, gestures or looks, and typically convey disparaging sentiments to people of color or other minority groups.
- Microaggressions have been shown in qualitative and quantitative studies to have detrimental effects on the mental health of minority groups.
- Patients are inherently vulnerable when they enter the clinical setting due to the power differential in the patient-physician interaction and are more susceptible to the negative effects of microaggressions.
- Physicians and residents, particularly those of color, women and LGBTQIA members, very frequently experience microaggressions from patients and their families and frequent biased encounters can be detrimental to mental health and work performance.

INTRODUCTION AND DEFINITIONS

"Again, one must not look for the gross and obvious. The subtle, cumulative miniassault is the substance of today's racism." Chester Pierce, *"Psychiatric Problems of the Black Minority"*[1]

The term microaggression was first coined in the 1970s by Harvard psychiatrist, Dr Chester Pierce, upon noting that his white students and colleagues often provided unsolicited feedback on his lesson plans and class structure. He noted:

"One could argue that I am hypersensitive, if not paranoid, about what must be an unusual kind of student-faculty dialogue…but what I know every black will understand, is that it is not what the student says in this dialogue, it is how he approaches me, how he talks to me, how he seems to regard me. Chester Pierce, Offensive Mechanisms[2]

It was from the accumulation of these subtle but demeaning interactions that the term microaggressions arose. They occur in everyday exchanges, are often delivered unconsciously either through words, tone, gestures or looks, and typically convey disparaging sentiments to people of color or other minority groups.[3]

The concept of microaggressions was revitalized and expanded upon in 2007 through the work of Columbia University clinical psychologists, Dr Derald Sue and colleagues, who further categorized microaggressions into three main subtypes: microassaults, microinsults, and microinvalidations **Table 1**.[3]

As defined by Sue and colleagues, microassaults are most like overt racism. Examples include using racial epithets like "oriental" or displaying a swastika. These are usually conscious and deliberate. They are only "micro" in that they are typically expressed in a private environment, although one could easily argue that there is no micro-component to this. Microinsults tend to be

University of Pennsylvania, Perelman School of Medicine, 235 South 8th Street, Philadelphia, PA 19106, USA
E-mail address: Michelle.weir@pennmedicine.upenn.edu

Dermatol Clin 41 (2023) 291–297
https://doi.org/10.1016/j.det.2022.08.006
0733-8635/23/

Table 1
Types of microaggressions

Type	Description
Microassults	Conscious, deliberate, verbal or non-verbal acts of bias or racism.
Microinsults	Subtle, unintentional comments that convey a demeaning message to the recipient. Often veiled as a compliment.
Microinvalidation	Biased statements that negate or nullify the feelings, thoughts, or experiences of a person of color.

more subtle but still convey a demeaning message to the recipient. They are often hidden as a "compliment." Examples include telling an Asian American that their English is very good or a Black man that he is very articulate or well spoken. Microinvalidations negate or nullify the feelings, thoughts or experiences of a person of color. Examples would include dismissing a biased interaction between a patient and a medical resident as "unintentional" or "misunderstood," or touting the self-ascribed virtue of being socially "color blind," which diminishes and ignores the impact race has on a person of color's experience in the United States.

Microaggressions all convey similar messages, which were subdivided by Sue into nine categories, but can be distilled down to (1) an ascription of "otherness" or not belonging to the majority social structure, (2) inferiority of personhood to that of the offender, (3) suggestion of criminality or propensity for violent behavior, and (4) invalidation of experience. They are derived from implicit personal, familial, or structural biases and cause harm by reinforcing traditional power differentials.[4]

IMPACT OF MICROAGGRESSIONS IN THE CLINICAL SETTING

As a single incident, a microaggression may seem harmless and easily dismissed as unintentional or a social misstep. The perception that this causes minimal harm is in defense of the offender, while overlooking the impact on the recipient, who has had to shoulder the burden of a lifetime of offenses. The cumulative effect is often likened to a turn of phrase "death by a thousand paper cuts," and has been shown in qualitative and quantitative studies to have detrimental effects on the mental health of minority groups. Experiencing racial microaggressions is linked to low self-esteem, stress, anxiety, depressive symptoms, and suicidal ideation.[5,6] Feelings of social isolation, helplessness, hopelessness, feeling judged, anger, and preoccupation are some of the psychological effects attributed to these experiences.[7] Although it is difficult to truly quantify its effect on mental health and wellbeing, understanding the impact of microaggressions on marginalized groups is "about listening to the voices of those most oppressed, ignored and silenced",[8] understanding their lived realities and giving this value.

Impact on Patients

In the clinical setting, there is naturally an unequal power differential between the patient and physician due to differences in the ill versus good state, medical knowledge, and sense of authority. In addition, physical or mental illness, while biological in nature, carries an emotional and psychological burden due to a loss of control, fear of prognosis, and financial stress, among many other potential stressors. Studies have also shown that Latinx, Asian, and Black patients often perceive medical staff as having judged them or treated them unfairly and believe that they have received worse medical care due to their race/ethnic group.[9] Thus, patients, particularly patients of color, are inherently vulnerable when they enter the clinical setting and are more susceptible to the effects of negative interactions. Microaggressions committed during these encounters can be of similar nature to those made in nonmedical settings; however, there are certain types of microaggressions that are more specific to clinical medicine. These include testimonial injustices and emotional microaggressions.

Testimonial injustices can occur when a patient's observation or story is not acknowledged or appreciated as having value by a physician due to conscious or unconscious prejudicial stereotypes about some facet of the patient's identity, whether that be race, gender, sexuality, class, age, or ability.[10] This is not to say that the patient's account of their illness should supersede medical or scientific knowledge, but the harm occurs when we allow our medical expertise, or worse, our unconscious biases, to silence the patient's narrative. This can manifest through poor face-to-face engagement during a consultation or dismissing or doubting patients' observations. We have all heard accounts from patients about the prior doctor who "just stared at their computer the whole time" or "didn't listen to a word I said." Testimonial injustices are more frequently experienced by black patients, who report poorer patient-physician communication than white patients including less nonverbal attention, empathy, and courtesy.[9,11] The harm caused by testimonial injustices includes devaluation of the patient's credibility in having knowledge of their own body as well as potential misdiagnoses by not adequately listening to the patient's story. A well-known example of the harm created by testimonial injustices is the racial disparity in maternal-infant health in the United States, with black women being three times more likely to die from pregnancy-related causes than white women regardless of socioeconomic factors.[12] Although the cause of this disparity is multifactorial and includes access to quality health care and underlying comorbid condition, implicit bias, and structural racism are acknowledged as contributing factors.[12] Numerous testimonies abound of pregnant, black women whose symptoms were ignored or discounted with perilous consequences.

Emotional microaggressions occur when physicians fail to consider or give credence to the emotional experiences of illness and disease.[10] They are "frequently motivated by assumptions about what constitutes appropriate emotional responses to medical symptoms and diagnoses and often compounded by stereotypes about emotions as they relate to race, sexuality, and especially to gender."[10] Illness can change the way patients view themselves and their relationship to the world. Physicians can commit a microaggression when we focus solely on the disease process and its management, and we don't take into consideration these existential consequences. In a memoir by Anatole Broyard, a man of mixed ethnicity of Louisiana-Creole decent, he recounts his experience with cancer and notes, "[t]o the typical physician, my illness is a routine incident in his rounds, whereas for me it is the crisis of my life. I would feel better if I had a doctor who at least perceived this incongruity.[13]"

A component of the patient–doctor relationship is to not only address the medical needs of a patient but also to provide emotional safety and comfort when navigating these difficult times. When a patient experiences a microaggression from their doctor or other health care provider it can be extremely devastating for a patient. Emotions associated with these experiences include anger, shame, betrayal, and disappointment. In addition, the emotional harm of not being heard in a setting that inherently requires trust often stays longer with the patient than the consequences of the medical diagnosis. Distrust that results from experiences of microaggressions in the clinical setting can ultimately contribute to decrease service utilization, reduced treatment compliance, and poorer physical and mental health.[10]

Mutual respect and open communication are important in avoiding microaggressions toward patients in the clinical setting. Physicians should be keenly aware that patients from marginalized groups have frequently had poor medical experiences. We should take note of our own potential biases then take the time to listen carefully to our patients, understand their illness as they experience it, and give credibility to their narrative.

Impact on Physicians and Medical Trainees

In recent years the impact of implicit bias and microaggressions on physicians and medical trainees has gained more attention. Physicians and residents, particularly those of color and women, very frequently experience these forms of bias from patients and their families. In a survey of over 800 physicians, 59% had a patient make an offensive remark about a personal characteristic, with the most common remarks being about age, ethnicity, gender, or race.[14] Almost half of the respondents have had patients request new physicians because of a personal characteristic.[14] A qualitative study conducted by Wheeler and colleagues[15] examined hospitalists' and internal medicine trainees' experience with bias in an academic medical center. Participants in the study reported that biased behavior ranged from refusal of care and microaggressions, to explicit racist, sexist and homophobic remarks and noted that biased interactions "take away from the ability to focus on training" and "make it harder to practice medicine. Residents are particularly susceptible to experiencing bias and microaggressions from patients as they are often perceived to have less authority yet have more frequent interactions with patients.

As evidenced by the prior subjective comments, frequent biased encounters can be detrimental to mental health and work performance. In fact, a study by Nadal and colleagues[16] showed that school or workplace microaggressions are most associated with traumatic stress symptoms. Although the study did not explore the potential reasons microaggressions in the educational or professional setting result in greater psychological distress, potential reasons include exacerbation of the imposter syndrome and the stereotype threat, both of which are rooted in structural bias. The imposter syndrome is a psychologic term that refers to the belief that one does not possess the skill, talent, or experiences necessary for a position, job or task, despite concrete evidence to the contrary. Although any individual may experience this phenomenon, it is mostly seen in people of color and women and can be a strong predictor of psychological distress and negatively affect career advancement.[17] The stereotype threat refers to the anxiety experienced by a member of a marginalized group, who knowing the negative stereotypes associated with their group, fears their actions could confirm those negative stereotypes. Both the imposter syndrome and the stereotype threat increase the emotional and cognitive burden of physicians and medical trainees of color, and repeated exposures to microaggressions can exacerbate those feeling leading to self-doubt, exhaustion, cynicism, and decreased performance.[15]

ADDRESSING MICROAGGRESSIONS IN THE CLINICAL SETTING

As previously mentioned, the harm from microaggressions does not come from a single act but from the accumulation of multiple acts and the psychological fatigue associated with its frequency. Given how impactful these experiences can be, what limits our ability to respond?

Often, as a recipient of a microaggression, there are multiple factors that come into play in one's decision to address the offense. First, there is the fear of being perceived as overreacting or hypersensitive. However, it is important to note, that this fear is derived from internalized structural biases that devalue the lived experience of marginalized peoples and is a form of testimonial injustice. Second, a decision needs to be made about the nature of the relationship between the offender and the recipient; is this a one-time encounter or is there a need or desire to maintain this relationship. Many people also feel that they do not know how to appropriately respond, whereas others may just be emotionally exhausted. Some psychologists refer to this exhaustion as the chronic state of "racial battle fatigue." When a microaggression is committed by a patient against a physician or other health care provider, the patient's clinical condition, fear of compromising the therapeutic alliance, and lack of institutional policies to support actions are other factors that contribute to one's decision for action.

Specifically looking at the clinical setting, microaggressions can be addressed using the ERASE framework that stands for EXPECT, RECOGNIZE, ADDRESS, SUPPORT, and ENCOURAGE.[18] The first component is to expect that these types of events will occur. A huge part of this step is taking the time to practice addressing a microaggression out loud. Practicing in advance allows you to better prepare yourself with specific language and techniques and can increase the likelihood that you will address the biased behavior when it occurs. The second part of the ERASE framework is RECOGNIZE. At the beginning of this article various types of microaggressions (microassaults, microinsults, microinvalidations) were defined. Understanding these definitions allows you to better recognize when they occur. The next component is to ADDRESS the biased event. This requires you first to take into consideration the context. In the clinical setting, you may ask yourself, "Is the patient mentally or physically stable?" If not, then addressing their behavior in that moment may not be ideal. Also take a moment to "take your own temperature." These types of interactions can invoke a sympathetic, "flight, fight or freeze" response and may impair critical thinking.[19] If you feel your anger rising, taking a pause or breath. Your tone and body language can convey as much as your words in both a helpful and harmful manner.

Specific Tactics for Addressing Microaggressions

When addressing a microaggression in the clinical setting perpetrated by a patient, it is important to maintain positive regard for your patient, as they often do not intend to be hurtful.[17] Focusing on the act and not the person is a helpful tip to avoid becoming defensive and responding with negative emotions. **Box 1** lists tactics for addressing microaggressions. Many of these tactics are most effective when used in combination and are outlined below.

One tactic for addressing a microaggression is to reflect the patient's biased statement back to them, often including a question, like "Can you explain that to me?" or "What is it about X that concerns you the most?" For example, I had a patient in clinic who came in to discuss his hair loss. He was explaining to me how he does not have a lot of money and so he must go to these "immigrant places" to get his

Box 1 **Tactics for addressing microaggressions[20]**
Inquire
Reflect
Reframe
"I" statements
Use preference statements
Re-direct
Revisit
Walk away

hair cut. When he completed his story, I stated back to him: "What I hear you saying is that you feel that your hair loss is related to having your hair cut by immigrants. I'm not sure I understand that connection, could you explain that to me?" He immediately back tracked and said, "Oh that didn't come out right. That's not what I meant." Reflecting shows understanding, reduces defensiveness, and helps the patient to become aware of their own statements. In most circumstances, patients can hear the bias in their own words and will correct their response. By coming from a place of curiosity you gain more information about a patient's perspective, and it opens the opportunity for dialogue, which in turn can strengthen the therapeutic alliance.[17]

Focusing on your own reaction to a patient's biased statement also helps to convey the impact of their words. This can be done by using "I" statements, which sounds non-threatening and takes the focus off the patient. "I felt uncomfortable when you referred to Asian people as Oriental. Asian is a more appropriate term." This can be followed by re-directing the conversation back to the clinical encounter. Another tactic is to express your corrective statement as a preference. "I prefer that we not talk about my personal appearance." Or "I prefer that you don't use the phrase 'that's so gay.' It makes it sound as if there is something wrong with being gay." Setting clear limits is also very important and framing it with preference statements such as "We don't use that kind of language in this clinic, so we prefer that you not use it either" helps to remove blame from the discussion and reduces defensiveness.

It is important for physicians and medical trainees to feel empowered to address and disarm a microaggression when it occurs. However, if you felt unprepared to respond to it in the moment consider revisiting it either later in that encounter or in a future encounter. This may be particularly important with patients with whom you expect to have a long-term therapeutic relationship. Leaving a microaggression unaddressed can have as negative an impact on the recipient as the microaggression itself.[18]

Finally, if a patient persistently shows abusive or discriminatory behavior it is reasonable for the physician or trainee to walk away from that encounter, ensuring that proper follow-up or transfer of care is in place. Of course, if an encounter ever feels unsafe or threatening then one should leave the room and notify security and risk management.

Creating a Supportive and Inclusive Culture

Returning to the ERASE framework, it is critically important to provide SUPPORT to those who experience a biased encounter by reflecting and debriefing with them. Failure to acknowledge it will often be interpreted as implicit acceptance. Simply expressing your own discomfort with the interaction can help build a safe environment for discussion. Allow the recipient of the aggression to express their own feelings and discuss how you or they might address a similar encounter in the future. The last component of the framework is to ENCOURAGE a positive culture. This should be a call to action that happens both at the individual and institutional level. This includes expressing openness to hearing concerns, instituting educational programming for trainees and faculty on addressing biased behavior, developing institutional reporting mechanisms, and identifying point people for support.

Responding When you Commit a Microaggression

As humans, we inherently have biases and are fallible. It is important to remember that despite our ethical values, we still hold unconscious biases that can contradict these values and make us susceptible to committing a microaggression. So, what steps can we take when we are the offenders? The suggestions outlined below are adapted from the ASSIST model (**Box 2**) proposed by Ackerman-Barger and colleagues.[21]

First, acknowledge your bias. Become familiar with your biases and actively take steps to mitigate them. This will help reduce the likelihood that you will commit a microaggression and that you will more quickly recognize and accept when you do.

Next, listen and accept feedback when a recipient responds to your comment. When confronted, avoid becoming defensive or responding in a manner that invalidates the recipient's experience of the microaggression. Understand that it is the impact of your words that matter at the moment, not your intention so take the opportunity to understand how your words have caused harm. Rather than experiencing the feedback as an attack on your moral character, see it as an opportunity to learn and grow as an individual. In line with that,

Box 2 ASSIST model
Acknowledge your bias
Seek feedback
Say you are sorry
Impact, not intent
Say, Thank you

thank the recipient for their courage in responding and taking the time to share their experience with you.

SUMMARY

Microaggressions will happen, and you will be, at various times, the recipient and the offender. It is important for us to recognize the inherent power differential that exists in the patient-physician relationship and the significant emotional harm and distrust that can be caused when we, as physicians, commit a microaggression against our patients. We must be conscious of our own biases and how they manifest during patient interactions, particularly when we are working with patients from historically marginalized populations and specifically when there is racial discordance. In a busy clinical setting, we will be prone to fall back on our "understanding" of certain demographics, but we must question whether those cognitive shortcuts are based on scientific evidence or our inherent biases. Actively identifying and working on diminishing our biases will help to reduce the incidence of these types of interactions.

Physicians and medical trainees, particularly those of color, women and LGBTQIA members, are increasingly the targets of microaggressions committed by patients. Learning to recognize and address microaggressions in the clinical setting creates a more supportive and inclusive environment for our patients, ourselves, and our trainees.

CLINICS CARE POINTS

- The ERASE framework (Expect, Recognize, Address, Support, Encourage) can be used to help guide responding to microaggressions.
- **Box 1** provides specific tactics for addressing microaggressions.
- The ASSIST model can help when you commit a microaggression.

DISCLOSURE

The author has no relevant disclosures.

REFERENCES

1. Pierce C. Psychiatric problems of the black minority. In: Arieti S, editor. American handbook of psychiatry I: the foundations of psychiatry. 2nd edition. New York: Basic Books; 1974. p. 512–23.

2. Pierce C. Offensive mechanism. In: Barbour F, editor. The black seventies. 1st edition. Boston: Porter Sargent; 1970. p. 265–82.

3. Sue D, Capodilupo C, Torino G, et al. Racial microaggressions in everyday life: implications for clinical practice. Am Pschologist 2007;62:271–86.

4. Williams M, Skinta M, Martin-Willett R. After pierce and sue: a revised racial microaggressions taxonomy. Perspect Pyschological Sci 2021;16(5):991–1007.

5. Spanierman LB, Clakr DA, Kim Y. Reviewing racial microaggressions research: documenting targets' experiences, harmful sequelae, and resistance strategies. Perspect Psychol Sci 2021;16(1):1037–59.

6. Farber R, Wedell E, Herchenroeder L, et al. Microaggressions and psychological health among college students: a moderated mediation model of rumination and social structure beliefs. J Racial Ethn Health Disparities 2021;8(1):245–55.

7. Hall JM, Fields B. "It's killing us!" Narrative of black adults about microaggression experiences and related health stress. Global Qual Nurs Res 2015;9(2):1–14.

8. Sue D. Microaggressions and "evidence": empirical or experiential reality? Perpectives Psychol Sci 2017;12(1):170–2.

9. Cooper LA, Beach MC, Johnson RL, et al. Delving below the surface. Understanding How Race Ethn Influence Relationships Health Care 2006;21(S1):S21–7.

10. Freeman L, Stewart H. Microaggressions in clinical medicine. Kennedy Inst Ethics J 2019;28(4):411–49.

11. Shen MJ, Peterson EB, Costas-Muniz R, et al. The effects of race and racial concordance on patient-physician communication: a systematic review of the literature. J Racial Ethn Health Disparities 2018;5(1):117–40.

12. Centers for Disease Control and Prevention. Working Together to Reduce Black Maternal Mortality. In: Health Equity Featured Articles. 2022. Available at: https://www.cdc.gov/healthequity/features/maternal-mortality/index.html?msclkid=ee88853cc71c11ecb36dbea763afbb93. Accessed April 30, 2022.

13. Broyard A. Intoxicated by my illness: and other writings on life and death. New York: C. Potter; 1992.

14. Medscape. Patient prejuidice: when credentials aren't enough. 2017. https://www.medscape.com/slideshow/2017-patient-prejudice-report-6009134?src=par_webmd_mscpmrk_patientprejudice&faf=1 (Accessed March 20, 2021).

15. Wheeler M, Bourmont S, Paul-Emile K, et al. Physician and trainee experiences with patient bias. JAMA Intern Med 2019;179(12):1678–85.

16. Nadal K, Erazo T, King R. Challenging definitions of psychological trauma: connecting racial microaggressions and traumatic stress. J Social Action Couns Psychol 2019;11(2):2–16.

17. LaDonna KA, Ginsburg S, Watling C. "Rising to the level of your incompetence": what physicians' self-assessment of their performance reveals about the imposter syndrome in medicine. Acad Med 2018; 93(5):763–8.

18. Goldenberg M, Cyrus K, Wilkins K. ERASE: a new framework for faculty to manage patient mistreatment of trainees. Acad Psychiatry 2019;43:396–9.

19. Wheeler DJ, Zapata J, Davis D, et al. Twelve Tips for responding to microaggressions and overt discrimination; When the patient offends the learner. Med Teach 2019;41(10):1112–7.

20. Adapted from UC Santa Cruz Academic Affairs. Tool: interrupting microaggression. Available at: https://academicaffairs.ucsc.edu/events/documents/Microaggressions_InterruptHO_2014_11_182v5.pdf. Accessed March 25, 2021.

21. Ackerman-Barger K, Jacobs N. The microaggressions triangle model: a humanistic approach to navigating microaggressions in health professions schools. Acad Med 2020;95(12S):S28–32.

Equity for Sexual and Gender Diverse Persons in Medicine and Dermatology

Julia L. Gao, MD[a,b,c,d],*, Kanika Kamal, BA[e], Klint Peebles, MD[f]

KEYWORDS

- Dermatology • Sexual diverse • Gender diverse • LGBTQ • Transgender • Hormone therapy
- Intersectionality • Cultural humility

KEY POINTS

- Incorporating sexual and gender diverse (SGD) health topics into dermatology training curricula and recruiting a diverse workforce inclusive of visible SGD-identified members of the health care team can improve the quality of dermatologic care for SGD patients.
- Collection of sexual orientation and gender identity data and its intersectionality with race and ethnicity is important for identifying and closing health disparity gaps.
- Delivery of culturally humble and affirming care for SGD individuals as well as advocacy for inclusive and validating public policy can improve dermatology outcomes for SGD patient populations.

INTRODUCTION

As the sexual and gender diverse (SGD) community continues to grow in the United States, the need for culturally competent and humble care will become an essential standard in dermatology practices. Nationwide surveys from 2021 suggest that almost 20 million US adults identify as SGD, doubling previous estimates from 2012, and estimates of the US transgender adult population have increased from 1.4 million to more than 2 million. This recent increase in SGD identification is likely multifactorial, reflecting the increased prevalence of such identities among younger US adult populations in addition to greater awareness and visibility of SGD identities, shifts in perceptions of safety and validation in the context of piecemeal legislative progress, and improved SGD-inclusive data collection.[1,2] However, compared with non-SGD individuals, SGD individuals experience disproportionately higher burdens of physical and/or psychosocial health conditions, including mental health issues and/or substance use.[3] They are more likely to have chronic health conditions, to lack access to health care, and, for women who have sex with women (WSW), less likely to receive cancer preventative care, such as breast and cervical cancer screening.[3] It is increasingly important for dermatologists to recognize that SGD patients also face dermatologic-specific disparities, with emerging research demonstrating increased prevalence of issues such as acne and alopecia in some transgender patients, increased risk of human immunodeficiency virus (HIV) infection and skin cancers in sexual minority men, increased incidence of human papillomavirus (HPV) infection in sexual minority women, and increased incidence of anal

[a] The Fenway Institute, Fenway Health, Boston, MA, USA; [b] Department of Dermatology, Beth Israel Deaconess Medical Center, 1340 Boylston Street, Boston, MA 02215, USA; [c] George Washington University School of Medicine & Health Sciences, Washington, DC, USA; [d] Dartmouth-Hitchcock Medical Center, One Medical Center Drive, Lebanon, NH 03766, USA; [e] Harvard Medical School, Harvard University, 25 Shattuck Street, Boston, MA 02115, USA; [f] Department of Dermatology, Kaiser-Permanente Mid-Atlantic Permanente Medical Group, 1221 Mercantile Lane, Largo, MD 20774, USA
* Corresponding author. Dartmouth-Hitchcock Medical Center, One Medical Center Drive, Lebanon, NH 03766
E-mail address: juliagao2022@gmail.com

Dermatol Clin 41 (2023) 299–308
https://doi.org/10.1016/j.det.2022.10.001
0733-8635/23/© 2022 Elsevier Inc. All rights reserved.

cancer and anal dysplasia in both men living with HIV infection who have sex with men (men who have sex with men [MSM]) and transgender women.[3-8] Dermatologists can play a key role in improving health equity for SGD patients through delivery of quality care, competent training, research, and advocacy efforts.

Definitions

Gender diverse refers to individuals whose gender identity or expression—which includes a spectrum ranging from man/masculine to woman/feminine, both, or neither—differs from their sex (male or female) assigned at birth; this may include transfeminine (ie, someone who was assigned male at birth but currently identifies as woman/feminine), transmasculine (ie, someone who was assigned female at birth but currently identifies as man/masculine), and gender nonconforming (ie, someone who does not adhere to any culturally defined gender norm, role, or identity) individuals (**Table 1**). Gender affirmation refers to the range of actions some individuals undertake to affirm their internal experience of gender identity or to better align their gender expression with their gender identity (**Fig. 1**).

Sexual diverse refers to individuals whose sexual identity, sexual orientation, or sexual behaviors differ from the presumed majority of the population. These individuals include those who identify as lesbian, gay, bisexual, pansexual, asexual, queer, or nonheterosexual (see **Table 1**). Individuals who are attracted to or have sexual contact with people of the same gender, such as MSM or WSW, also fall under this umbrella term. The concept of sexual orientation refers to the individual one is drawn to romantically, emotionally, and sexually.[9]

A person's sexual orientation identity is independent of their gender identity. In fact, an individual may have different sexual and romantic or emotional orientations. For example, someone may be sexually attracted to more than one gender, but they might only be able to envision themselves in a romantic relationship with someone of the same gender. Finally, a person's expressed sexual orientation identity and attraction does not necessarily predict behavior. Dermatologists should ask specific questions in the appropriate clinically relevant context and avoid making assumptions about behavior based on identity and vice-versa.

DISCUSSION
Curricula Inclusiveness in Dermatology Education

It is clear that dermatologists must be prepared to provide care for SGD populations, yet the incorporation of SGD-specific curricula in both medical school and dermatology residency training remains lacking.[10-12] A survey of 123 graduate medical education dermatology residency programs demonstrated a gap between desired and current education in SGD care. Although 80% of dermatology program directors believed that training in SGD care is important for trainees, most programs dedicated little time for SGD training in the curricula, with 46% of programs dedicating zero curricular hours and 37% dedicating only 1 to 2 hours to covering SGD care. The most frequently cited barriers to SGD-content integration were lack of time in the curriculum schedule (69%) and lack of experienced faculty (62%).[13]

This study also revealed a lack of consistency in which SGD health-related topics were discussed. The most frequently addressed topic was dermatologic concerns secondary to HIV/AIDS (73%), which risks further stigmatizing already marginalized populations when this is the only SGM-related education provided during training. Few programs (12%) covered SGM-oriented history taking and physical examination skills. Other SGD-related topics addressed included pronoun use (26%), skin cancer risk in sexual diverse patients (24%), and the cutaneous effects of gender-affirming hormone therapy (18%).[13] Such coverage is often insufficient for delivering quality care to SGD patients. Rather than emphasizing *cultural competency*, which implies there is a teachable categorical knowledge about a group of people and assumes that there is an endpoint to becoming fully competent, efforts should focus on cultivating *cultural humility*, which involves an ongoing process of self-critique combined with an interpersonal willingness to learn from others.[14,15]

Incorporating SGD-related health topics into existing Accreditation Council for Graduate Medical Education (ACGME) core competencies and dermatology resident assessments, recruiting diverse, SGD-identifying faculty interested in SGD dermatology, blending SGD content into didactic curricula, and creating a welcoming environment for both SGD patients as well as SGD trainees are keys to creating the next generation of dermatologists that will mitigate these health disparities.[10] Other steps that dermatologists and trainees should take include engaging in SGD dermatology educational sessions in conferences and other educational forums and reviewing the newly released SGD-focused module for the American Academy of Dermatology (AAD) Basic Dermatology Curriculum. Most importantly, all stakeholders in curricula development must be

Table 1
A relevant but nonexhaustive list of sexual and gender diverse–related terminology

Terminology	Definition
Gender identity	A person's internal sense of self as masculine/man, feminine/woman, a blend of both, neither, or another gender. *Note: a person's gender identity may or may not align with their sex assigned at birth*
Gender expression	A person's external display of their gender identity (eg, through clothing, grooming, behavior, speech, and so forth)
Gender affirmation	Refers to decisions, behaviors, or interventions that affirm an individual's gender identity. Domains may include psychological/self, social, legal, medical, and surgical affirmation. Particularly in the surgical and medical context, these steps may be referred to as "transitioning." Not all gender diverse people will desire all or any of these domains of affirmation.
Gender dysphoria	Clinically significant distress caused when a person's assigned sex at birth does not align with their gender identity
Sex assigned at birth	The sex attributed to an individual at the time of their birth, most often based on observation of external anatomy
AFAB	Assigned female at birth
AMAB	Assigned male at birth
Cisgender	An individual whose gender identity and expression align with the typical expectations of their sex assigned at birth
Gender diverse	An individual whose gender identity and expression differ from their sex assigned at birth
Transfeminine	An individual who was assigned male at birth but currently identifies as feminine. Some also use the term transgender woman, trans woman, or MTF
Transmasculine	An individual who was assigned female at birth but currently identifies as masculine. Some also use the term transgender man, trans man, or FTM
Genderqueer	An umbrella term for gender identities that differ from the binary identities of male and female. This includes people who view themselves as a combination of both male and female, neither male nor female, different gender at different times, or no specific gender at all
Gender nonconforming	An individual who does not adhere to any one particular gender norm, role, or identity. Can include gender fluid, androgynous, two-spirit, or more
Nonbinary	Gender identities other than the traditional female and male binary identities
Genderfluid	An individual who views themselves as male, female, or nonbinary at different times or under different circumstances
Agender	An individual who identifies as having no gender
Intersex	An individual born with any number of sex characteristics, including chromosomes and gonads, that do not fit typical binary notions of expectations of male and female bodies. Also known as "variations of sex characteristics" and "differences of sex development"
Sexual orientation identity	A person's inherent pattern of emotional, romantic, and/or sexual attraction (or lack of attraction) to other people. *Note: a person's sexual orientation is independent of their gender identity*
Heterosexual/Straight	An individual who is emotionally or sexually attracted to people of the opposite sex or gender

(continued on next page)

Table 1
(continued)

Terminology	Definition
Sexual diverse	An individual whose sexual identity, sexual orientation, or sexual behaviors differ from the presumed majority of the population
Gay	An individual who is emotionally or sexually attracted to people of the same sex or gender
MSM	Men who have sex with men
WSW	Women who have sex with women
Lesbian	A woman who is emotionally or sexually attracted to women. *Note: some women may also identify as being gay*
Bisexual	An individual who is emotionally or sexually attracted to both men and women
Pansexual	An individual who is emotionally or sexually attracted to any sex or gender
Demisexual	An individual who does not experience primary sexual attraction but may experience secondary sexual attraction after forming a close emotional connection
Asexual	An individual who does not experience sexual attraction toward individuals of any energy. *Note: may or may not be emotionally or romantically attracted to others*
Romantic orientation	An individual's pattern of romantic attraction based on a person's gender regardless or one's sexual orientation

Abbreviations: FTM, female to male; MTF, male to female.

explicit and intentional with the integration of SGD content. SGD curricula do not have to include exclusively de novo content; in fact, interweaving SGD-related concepts organically into the existing curriculum allows SGD health to be seen as integral rather than supplemental. Curricula amendments can simply include reframing existing patient vignettes to include diverse relationships, behaviors, and identities. For example, when teaching about isotretinoin, a case framed around a transgender patient can teach cultural humility without compromising the quality of the learning achieved from a module with a cisgender patient.

Workforce Diversity

Workforce diversity is critical for an assembly of physicians molded by diverse lived experiences to improve care for all populations.[16,17] It is associated with increased patient trust, satisfaction, and adherence to medical advice.[16] Exposure to SGD patients and colleagues in medical training reduces anti-SGD bias among medical professionals, which is especially important, as SGD individuals face disproportionate stigmatization, discrimination, and mistreatment when accessing health care services.[18] Yet, SGD trainees continue to report fears of discrimination in medical school

and residency applications, higher levels of mistreatment during medical training, and discrimination from both colleagues and patients, all of which limits their visibility.[10,16,19]

For the first time in 2020, the AAD Member Satisfaction Survey included questions about sexual orientation and gender identity (SOGI). A secondary analysis revealed that 3.7% of respondents identify as SGD, more so among male (6.7%) compared with female respondents (1.0%), and only 0.3% identify as transgender. In contrast to the 2021 Gallup survey where 9.5% of women and 5.4% of men identify as SGD, these data suggest that SGD women may be underrepresented among US dermatologists.[2,20] This underrepresentation is also present in the training pipeline, as dermatology has the lowest percentage of SGD female graduating medical students among all medical specialties (1.9%)[21]; this highlights a need for dermatology residency training programs to explicitly prioritize SGD identities in recruitment efforts to cultivate a visibly diverse and inclusive workforce.[20]

Compared with non-SGD dermatologists, SGD dermatologists were more likely to be male, younger, and practice in academic settings. Although most SGD dermatologists who responded were open about their sexual orientation at home and with work colleagues, only

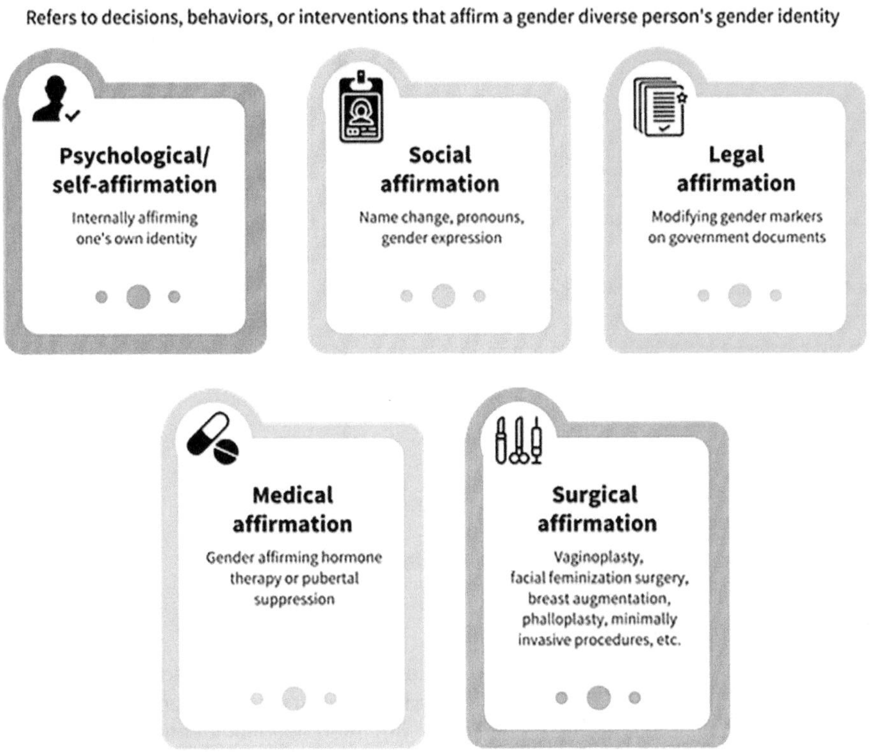

Refers to decisions, behaviors, or interventions that affirm a gender diverse person's gender identity

Psychological/ self-affirmation

Internally affirming one's own identity

Social affirmation

Name change, pronouns, gender expression

Legal affirmation

Modifying gender markers on government documents

Medical affirmation

Gender affirming hormone therapy or pubertal suppression

Surgical affirmation

Vaginoplasty, facial feminization surgery, breast augmentation, phalloplasty, minimally invasive procedures, etc.

Fig. 1. Domains of gender affirmation.

48% were open about their sexual orientation with patients.[20] Institutions should partner with diversity offices and SGD community organizations to foster learning and practice environments that signal unconditional support of their SGD students and employees. Steps to creating such environments include development of safe spaces as well as efforts to highlight SGD faculty and mentorship programs. These simple steps not only have the potential to affect the motivation and mental health of health care workers and trainees but also through reducing burnout can improve patient outcomes and promote SGD provider visibility.

Sexual Orientation and Gender Identity Data Collection

The systematic and routine collection of SOGI data is essential to identifying SGD patients and their health needs, delivering high-quality affirming therapeutic interventions, and implementing legislative and regulatory policies to address SGD health care disparities.[22–24] However, the rate of demographic data collection on SGD patients in dermatology research remains essentially nonexistent for the last 10 years despite numerous calls to action.[25] Multiple studies have demonstrated that most of the patients, including those who identify as cisgender and heterosexual, are amenable to answering SOGI questions, which should be included in standard patient registration forms and electronic health records.[22,26–28] SOGI data collection should also be standardized in all trainee and physician workforce surveys to better identify SGD providers and subsequently tailor outreach and support to close diversity gaps.[20] Clinical trials should also optimize enrollment of underrepresented minorities, including SGD patients, through use of SOGI questions rather than the current male/female binary for classifying trial participants.[29,30]

A 2-step approach should be used to measure gender identity by asking for self-reported assigned sex at birth and current gender identity (**Fig. 2**).[30,31] In addition, accurately recording a person's name and pronouns without labeling either as *preferred* or *chosen* is necessary to improve culturally competent care for transgender and gender diverse patients.[30] It is also important to routinely confirm and update SOGI data, as identities may be dynamic across the life span.

There is no uniform consensus on how to ask for identification of gender identity. Presented here is one example of how gender identity can be elicited through an inclusive, 2-step method, based on recent literature.[30]

1. What best matches your current gender identity?
   (Check all that apply)
   ☐ Man
   ☐ Woman
   ☐ Genderqueer or gender fluid
   ☐ Non-binary or not exclusively man or woman
   ☐ Questioning or exploring
   ☐ None of these describe me (please elaborate: _____)
   ☐ Prefer not to answer

2. What was your assigned sex at birth?
   (Meaning the gender marker that appears on your original birth certificate)
   (Choose one)
   ☐ Male
   ☐ Female
   ☐ Intersex or variation of sex characteristics
   ☐ None of these describe me (please elaborate: _____)
   ☐ Prefer not to answer

Fig. 2. Two-step approach for identifying gender identity.

Intersectionality

Drawing on black feminist and critical legal theory, legal scholar Kimberlé Crenshaw coined the term "intersectionality" to describe the multiple social forces and ideological instruments through which power and disadvantage are expressed and legitimized, including how systems of oppression overlap to create distinct lived experiences for people with multiple minority identity categories.[32] Intersectionality within the SGD community and the disparities among subgroups within the community have been understudied. Understanding how other aspects of identity—including race, ethnicity, culture, language, religion, socioeconomic status, and ability, among others—integrate with SGD identity is crucial to fully characterize inequities and work toward actionable change through research, clinical care, and policy action. For example, the experiences of a white gay man from middle-class suburbia are likely to be vastly different from that of a transgender Native American woman living in an impoverished rural setting. These wider inequities have been briefly characterized for SGD patients of color.[33] A qualitative study of 39 transgender patients of color reported that 82% of participants sought out SGD-friendly health care locations in an effort to avoid discrimination but still feared racism, with a majority believing that they would have received better treatment if they were cisgender or white. Some also reported reluctance to reveal their gender identity to providers of their own race due to fear of transphobia.[34] Researchers and trainees must dedicate attention to studying the intersectionality of these identities. In addition, dermatology residency programs must prioritize recruiting trainees with intersectional identities to better serve these communities.

Advocating for Sexual and Gender Diverse Patients

Advocacy in daily practice

Being an advocate can be as simple as treating SGD patients with respect, which has been associated with significantly lower prevalence of suicidal ideation and attempts in transgender patients.[35] Using the correct name and pronouns for SGD individuals shows appropriate respect, reduces gender dysphoria, avoids unnecessary distress from "deadnaming" a patient (defined as the act of calling an individual by their birth name when they have changed their name as part of gender affirmation), and prevents unintentional disclosure to others. When first meeting a patient, avoid language that assumes gender identity (eg, sir, ma'am, Ms/Mr/Mrs) until the patient identifies their gender and preferred pronouns.[36,37] If unsure, simply ask the patient for their pronouns; this can be normalized in conversations by providing your pronouns first and by including SOGI questions on patient intake forms. Ensuring accurate documentation in the patient's medical record helps prevent misgendering of the patient by other members of the care team.

Advocacy can also take the form of adopting inclusive, nonassuming, and nongendered language into the history and physical examination process. For example, when understanding a patient's risk of conditions such as HIV infection, HPV infection, squamous cell carcinoma, syphilis, and other dermatologic issues, it is important to take a thorough, gender-inclusive sexual history for *all* patients and to avoid operating on assumptions (**Fig. 3**). Such language would include using terms such as "people who can become pregnant" rather than "women who can become pregnant." Instead of using language that assumes the patient has an opposite sex partner, such as "do you have a husband?," ask "are you in a relationship?"[36] Further, it is important to use nongendered language when asking about a patient's anatomy or "organ inventory" (**Fig. 4**).

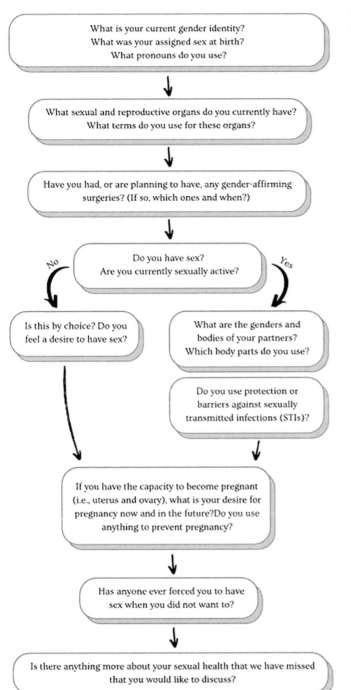

Fig. 3. Inclusive sexual and gender history language and algorithm.

What is your current gender identity?
What was your assigned sex at birth?
What pronouns do you use?

What sexual and reproductive organs do you currently have?
What terms do you use for these organs?

Have you had, or are planning to have, any gender-affirming surgeries? (If so, which ones and when?)

Do you have sex?
Are you currently sexually active?

No / Yes

Is this by choice? Do you feel a desire to have sex?

What are the genders and bodies of your partners? Which body parts do you use?

Do you use protection or barriers against sexually transmitted infections (STIs)?

If you have the capacity to become pregnant (i.e., uterus and ovary), what is your desire for pregnancy now and in the future? Do you use anything to prevent pregnancy?

Has anyone ever forced you to have sex when you did not want to?

Is there anything more about your sexual health that we have missed that you would like to discuss?

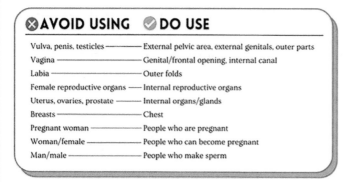

Fig. 4. Inclusive sexual health language.

The importance of inclusive, nongendered language further extends to the way dermatologists describe aesthetic and gender-affirming procedures. Historically, dermatologists have relied on the terms "feminine" and "masculine" to describe traditional aesthetic ideals and beauty. Yet, many cisgender and SGD patients may reject such labels, and this language may worsen gender dysphoria. Rather than asking patients if they would like a masculine jawline or a feminine brow and forehead region, use specific language to describe certain features (eg, "convex, projected cheek contour") and provide points of contrast to help patients identify and meet their goals.[38] If after starting the encounter with inclusive language a patient then desires to use gendered terms, follow their lead. Finally, although no health care provider wants to say the wrong thing, this sometimes leads to avoidance of acknowledging SGD patients, which may irreparably undermine rapport. SGD patients present to dermatology because they have a skin issue to be addressed, and an accidental misstep can be rectified by a contrite apology with return of focus to the main issue at hand: their dermatologic needs.

Potential questions to ask an individual about their sexual history and behaviors in an inclusive manner.

Legislative and regulatory advocacy

More than 300 anti-SGD bills have been introduced in states across the country in 2022 at the time of this writing.[39] Dozens of these bills target transgender people and their ability to seek medical care, and dermatology will be significantly affected if these discriminatory measures are implemented.

In February 2022, the governor of Texas issued an order restricting access to gender-affirming medical care for transgender youth and classified such cases as "child abuse." As of March 2022, at least 15 states have already followed suit and

implemented or are currently considering laws that restrict access to gender-affirming care, affecting more than 58,000 transgender youth and young adults.[40] Each of these bills would either criminalize health care providers who provide gender-affirming care to minors or subject them to discipline from licensing boards. Ten of these states would allow civil suits for damages to be filed against medical providers who violate these proposed laws. Finally, half of these bills would bar certain insurance providers from covering gender-affirming care.[40] Depending on the specific language of each state's law, dermatologists may be prevented from delivering important gender-affirming care, including preoperative and perioperative hair removal, scar revision, minimally invasive facial and body modification, and other procedures. Dermatologists have been successful advocates for their patients in recent years, with the notable example of pushing for the adoption of gender-neutral language in the Food and Drug Administration–mandated Risk Evaluation and Mitigation Strategies program for isotretinoin, iPLEDGE. Especially with the latest series of legislative assaults on transgender people, physicians must use their platforms of knowledge, privilege, and power to amplify the voices of our most silenced SGD communities and to reassure our patients that the medical community is, and will always remain, the greatest champion and advocate for SGD health and well-being.

SUMMARY

Dermatologists can play a key role in improving health care equity for SGD patients through improving awareness of sexual and gender diverse identities that may impact skin health, building SGD-inclusive curricula and environments in medical training, promoting workforce diversity, practicing with intersectionality in mind, and engaging in patient advocacy across the policy spectrum.

CLINICS CARE POINTS

- To enhance SGD curricula inclusiveness in dermatology, programs should be intentional about integrating this content into both didactic and clinical education.

- Student and trainee diversity in dermatology is crucial for SGD patient trust, satisfaction, and adherence to medical advice. Improving SGD trainee visibility includes recruiting trainees who identify across the spectrum of SGD identities as well as institutional partnership with diversity offices and the broader SGD community.

- SOGI data collection is essential for providers to properly deliver high-quality, affirming health care to SGD patients. In addition, SOGI collection in dermatology clinical trials will ensure that the risks and benefits incurred by participating in novel drug trials are distributed equitably across various marginalized populations.

- Intersectionality is understudied despite a growing body of SGD dermatology literature and is crucial to fully characterize inequities within SGD subgroups so that actionable change may occur through research, clinical care, and policy action. Recruitment of trainees in dermatology with intersectional identities is of utmost importance to diversify the workforce pipeline.

- Advocacy is an important component of care for underserved populations, including SGD individuals, particularly when legislation and other policy initiatives directly threaten the ability of physicians to provide unbiased and lifesaving care. Dermatologists can engage in advocacy by simply validating patient identities in their daily practices and also by championing legislative equality for SGD people at the local, state, and federal levels.

DISCLOSURE

The authors have no commercial or financial conflicts of interest or disclosures to report.

REFERENCES

1. Foundation HRC. We are here: understanding the size of the LGBTQ+ community. 2022. Available at: https://hrc-prod-requests.s3-us-west-2.amazonaws.com/We-Are-Here-120821.pdf. Accessed March 30, 2022.

2. LGBT identification in U.S. ticks up to 7.1%. gallup. 2022. Available at: https://news.gallup.com/poll/389792/lgbt-identification-ticks-up.aspx. Accessed March 30, 2022.

3. Yeung H, Luk KM, Chen SC, et al. Dermatologic care for lesbian, gay, bisexual, and transgender persons: epidemiology, screening, and disease prevention. J Am Acad Dermatol 2019;80(3):591–602.

4. Gao JL, King DS, Modest AM, et al. Acne risk in transgender and gender diverse populations: a retrospective comparative cohort study. J Am Acad Dermatol 2022;S0190-9622(22):00394–402.

5. Thoreson N, Grasso C, Potter J, et al. Incidence and factors associated with androgenetic alopecia among transgender and gender-diverse patients treated with masculinizing hormone therapy. JAMA Dermatol 2021;157(3):348–9.

6. Silverberg MJ, Lau B, Justice AC, et al. Risk of anal cancer in HIV-infected and HIV-uninfected individuals in North America. Clin Infect Dis 2012;54(7):1026–34.

7. Kobayashi T, Sigel K, Gaisa M. Prevalence of anal dysplasia in HIV-infected transgender women. Sex Transm Dis 2017;44(11):714.

8. Ruanpeng D, Chariyalertsak S, Kaewpoowat Q, et al. Cytological anal squamous intraepithelial lesions associated with anal high-risk human papillomavirus infections among men who have sex with men in northern Thailand. PloS one 2016;11(5):e0156280.

9. Campaign HR. Sexual orientation and gender identity definition. Human Rights Campaign; 2019.

10. Sternhell-Blackwell K, Mansh M, Peebles JK. Residency education on sexual and gender minority health: ensuring culturally competent dermatologists and excellent patient care. JAMA Dermatol 2020;156(5):497–9.

11. Zelin NS, Hastings C, Beaulieu-Jones BR, et al. Sexual and gender minority health in medical curricula in new England: a pilot study of medical student comfort, competence and perception of curricula. Med Education Online 2018;23(1):1461513.

12. Obedin-Maliver J, Goldsmith ES, Stewart L, et al. Lesbian, gay, bisexual, and transgender–related content in undergraduate medical education. Jama 2011;306(9):971–7.

13. Jia JL, Nord KM, Sarin KY, et al. Sexual and gender minority curricula within US dermatology residency programs. JAMA Dermatol 2020;156(5):593–4.

14. Stubbe DE. Practicing cultural competence and cultural humility in the care of diverse patients. Focus 2020;18(1):49–51.

15. Khan S. Cultural Humility vs. Cultural Competence — and Why Providers Need Both. Bostom Medical Center Health System. Available at: https://healthcity.bmc.org/policy-and-industry/cultural-humility-vs-cultural-competence-providers-need-both. Accessed May 1, 2022, 2022.

16. Mansh M, Garcia G, Lunn MR. From patients to providers: changing the culture in medicine toward sexual and gender minorities. Acad Med 2015;90(5):574–80.

17. Street RL, O'Malley KJ, Cooper LA, et al. Understanding concordance in patient-physician relationships: personal and ethnic dimensions of shared identity. Ann Fam Med 2008;6(3):198–205.

18. Ayhan CHB, Bilgin H, Uluman OT, et al. A systematic review of the discrimination against sexual and gender minority in health care settings. Int J Health Serv 2020;50(1):44–61.

19. Mansh M, White W, Gee-Tong L, et al. Sexual and gender minority identity disclosure during undergraduate medical education:"in the closet" in medical school. Acad Med 2015;90(5):634–44.

20. Mansh MD, Dommasch E, Peebles JK, et al. Lesbian, gay, bisexual, and transgender identity and disclosure among dermatologists in the US. JAMA Dermatol 2021;157(12):1512–4.

21. Mori WS, Gao Y, Linos E, et al. Sexual orientation diversity and specialty choice among graduating allopathic medical students in the United States. JAMA Netw open 2021;4(9):e2126983.

22. Streed CG Jr, Grasso C, Reisner SL, et al. Sexual orientation and gender identity data collection: clinical and public health importance. Washington, DC: American Public Health Association; 2020. p. 991–3.

23. Schabath MB, Curci MB, Kanetsky PA, et al. Ask and tell: the importance of the collection of sexual orientation and gender identity data to improve the quality of cancer care for sexual and gender minorities. J Oncol Pract 2017;13(8):542–6.

24. Cahill S, Makadon H. Sexual orientation and gender identity data collection in clinical settings and in electronic health records: a key to ending LGBT health disparities. LGBT health 2014;1(1):34–41.

25. Boothby-Shoemaker W, Mansh M, Sternhell-Blackwell K, et al. Sexual orientation and gender identity inclusion in dermatology research: a ten-year analysis. J Am Acad Dermatol 2022;S0190-9622(22):00534–5.

26. Cahill S, Singal R, Grasso C, et al. Do ask, do tell: high levels of acceptability by patients of routine collection of sexual orientation and gender identity data in four diverse American community health centers. PloS one 2014;9(9):e107104.

27. Rullo JE, Foxen JL, Griffin JM, et al. Patient acceptance of sexual orientation and gender identity questions on intake forms in outpatient clinics: a pragmatic randomized multisite trial. Health Serv Res 2018;53(5):3790–808.

28. Ruben MA, Kauth MR, Meterko M, et al. Veterans' reported comfort in disclosing sexual orientation and gender identity. Med Care 2021;59(6):550–6.

29. Price KN, Alavi A, Hsiao JL, et al. Gender minority patients in dermatology clinical trials. Int J Women's Dermatol 2020;6(5):438.

30. Kronk CA, Everhart AR, Ashley F, et al. Transgender data collection in the electronic health record: current concepts and issues. J Am Med Inform Assoc 2022;29(2):271–84.

31. Group G. Best practices for asking questions to identify transgender and other gender minority respondents on population-based surveys. Los Angeles, CA: eScholarship, University of California; 2014.

32. Crenshaw KW. On intersectionality: essential writings. New York, NY: The New Press; 2017.

33. Ruoss AV, Short WR, Kovarik CL. The patient's perspective: reorienting dermatologic care for lesbian, gay, bisexual, transgender, and queer/questioning patients. Dermatol Clin 2020;38(2):191–9.

34. Howard SD, Lee KL, Nathan AG, et al. Healthcare experiences of transgender people of color. J Gen Intern Med 2019;34(10):2068–74.

35. Herman JL, Brown TN, Haas AP. Suicide thoughts and attempts among transgender adults: Findings from the 2015 US Transgender Survey. 2019.

36. National LGBT Health Education Center TFI. Providing Inclusive Services and Care for LGBT People: A Guide for Health Care Staff. 2016. Available at: https://www.lgbtqiahealtheducation.org/wp-content/uploads/Providing-Inclusive-Services-and-Care-for-LGBT-People.pdf

37. Krempasky C, Harris M, Abern L, et al. Contraception across the transmasculine spectrum. Am J Obstet Gynecol 2020;222(2):134–43.

38. Beuttler M, MacGregor J. A genderfluid approach to aesthetic language in dermatology. J Drugs Dermatol JDD 2022;21(1):96–9.

39. Human Rights Campaign. ICYMI: As lawmakers escalate attacks on transgender youth across the country, some GOP leaders stand up for transgender youth. 2022. Available at: https://www.hrc.org/press-releases/icymi-as-lawmakers-escalate-attacks-on-transgender-youth-across-the-country-some-gop-leaders-stand-up-for-transgender-youth. Accessed April 37, 2022.

40. Conron KJ, O'Neill K, Vasquez LA. Prohibiting gender-affirming medical care for youth. 2021. Available at: https://williamsinstitute.law.ucla.edu/publications/bans-trans-youth-health-care/

The Social Determinants of Health and Their Impact on Dermatologic Health, Part 1

The Social Determinants of Health and Their Dermatologic Implications

Sacharitha Bowers, MD[a],*, Aileen Y. Chang, MD[b]

KEYWORDS

- Social determinants of health • Structural determinants of health • Dermatologic health disparities

KEY POINTS

- The social determinants of health (SDoH) are nonmedical factors that greatly influence the health and well-being of individuals, across every discipline in medicine, including dermatology.
- Improving dermatologic health outcomes requires an understanding of the structural and SDoH, how the SDoH affect dermatologic health and lead to disparities in patients with dermatologic disorders.
- Atopic dermatitis, psoriasis, hidradenitis suppurativa, and melanoma are among the conditions that have growing evidence on the influence of the SDoH on dermatologic health.
- The implications of the SDoH on dermatologic health include disparities in disease prevalence, severity, diagnosis, treatment, and patient outcomes.

INTRODUCTION

In recent years, there has been renewed commitment to health equity—the ability of every individual to attain their "full health potential" and not be "disadvantaged from achieving this potential due to social position or other socially determined circumstances".[1] Our collective understanding around what shapes the health and well-being of individuals, communities, and entire populations has evolved over time, largely due to an improved understanding of the factors outside an individual's control—namely, the social determinants of health (SDoH), defined as *the conditions in which people are born, grow, live, learn, work, play, and age*.[2,3] More recent evidence has shown that SDoH affect health disparities and health outcomes to a far greater degree than access to health care alone.[4,5] The United States (US), despite being among the wealthiest countries in the world, suffers from worse infant mortality, chronic disease burden, and life expectancy, compared with similarly wealthy nations.[6] Research shows that investment in the SDoH can lead to positive health outcomes and a reduction in overall health spending.[7]

SDoH can negatively affect patients with cutaneous pathologic condition across a variety of conditions, which has resulted in widening dermatologic health disparities. Dermatologists must become aware of how nonmedical factors influence the daily lives and health outcomes of our

a Division of Dermatology, Department of Internal Medicine, Loyola University Medical Center, Stritch School of Medicine, 1S260 Summit Ave, Oakbrook Terrace, IL 60181, USA; b Department of Dermatology, University of California San Francisco, Zuckerberg San Francisco General Hospital, 995 Potrero Avenue, Building 90, Ward 92, San Francisco, CA 94110, USA
* Corresponding author.
E-mail address: sachbow@gmail.com

Dermatol Clin 41 (2023) 309–316
https://doi.org/10.1016/j.det.2022.10.002
0733-8635/23/© 2022 Elsevier Inc. All rights reserved.

derm.theclinics.com

patients to be well equipped to fully meet patients' health needs and decrease health disparities. Advancing health equity is fundamentally predicated on a reduction in health and health-care disparities, which require understanding and addressing the SDoH. Part 1 of this 2-part series aims to provide dermatology practitioners and trainees with a thorough understanding of the SDoH and how they affect dermatologic disease and health outcomes; Part 2 will address interventions that can be taken to modify their harmful influences on health.

Social Determinants of Health

For centuries, the health effects of resource deprivation, such as lack of food, clean water, sanitation, and shelter, have been a part of public health discourse.[8] Although earlier literature focused primarily on the relationship between poverty and health, a growing body of work has examined the complex interplay between broad social, economic, and political factors that affect health. The SDoH are defined as *the conditions in which people are born, grow, work, live, learn, work, play, and age*, and are considered to be nonmedical factors that influence and determine health outcomes.[2,3] They encompass the social, economic, and political conditions that affect the daily lives and health of individuals and their communities.[2]

It is clear that greater social disadvantage is associated with overall poorer health.[9] A meta-analysis by Galea and colleagues[10] revealed that in 2000, the number of deaths in the United States attributable to low education, racial segregation, low social support, poverty, and income equality was comparable to deaths from the leading pathophysiological causes of acute myocardial infarction, cerebrovascular disease, and lung cancer. Of note, medical care determines only about 15% to 20% of an individual's health. The remainder 80% to 85% of a person's health is determined by biology/genetics, behavior, social, environmental, and physical influences, with the largest component of this being the SDoH.[4,5] Consequently, improving health outcomes and reducing health disparities necessitates a prioritization of the SDoH, which are composed of 5 main categories[3] and can affect health in a multitude of complex and intersecting ways,[9,11,12] with examples described in **Table 1**.[3,11,13]

Structural Determinants of Health

Fully understanding and addressing SDoH requires attention to their upstream systems and structures, known as the *structural determinants of health*. These upstream factors include governance, economic, social and public policies, and cultural and societal values that generate and maintain socioeconomic status (SES). The structural determinants of health influence the distribution of a society's resources and, along with gender, race, and ethnicity, determine the downstream SDoH.[14,15]

It is the structural determinants of health that dictate the systems and policies that determine access to clean air and water, affordable and safe housing, nutritious food, job opportunities with nontoxic working environments, and safe neighborhoods and communities, with access to quality schools, parks, and health care. The causal pathways linking upstream structural determinants with downstream social determinants, and ultimately with health effects and outcomes, are long, complex and multifactorial, making the structural determinants harder to study and address.[11,16] However, failing to look upstream fails to address the deeply rooted causes of health disparities and further jeopardizes improving health equity.

Socioeconomic Status

Socioeconomic status (SES) is defined as the social standing or class of an individual or group and ideally is measured by multiple constructs, including education, income, occupation,[17] and wealth.[4] SES is closely linked to racial and ethnic disparities because minoritized racial-ethnic groups are disproportionately represented in lower SES groups. According to the US Census Bureau, Black and Hispanic populations in 2019 consisted a greater share of those living in poverty than any other racial and ethnic group, and in numbers that were disproportionately high relative to their representation in the general population.[18] Low SES position is correlated with worse health.[11] Numerous evidence links low SES to adverse health risks and worse health outcomes, such as lead ingestion through substandard housing with resulting neurological and physical development[19,20] and exposure to pollutants and allergens in low-income neighborhoods leading to asthma exacerbations.[21,22]

The Role of Racism

Although at one time racism was considered an independent social determinant of health, the evidence is clear that it is an underlying structural determinant of health that permeates all the SDoH and is a primary driver of systemic inequity. Understanding how structural and SDoH influence health outcomes requires examination of the

Table 1
Social determinants of health: categories, definitions, examples of health impact

SDoH	Definition	Example of Health Impact
Education access and quality	The connection of education to health and well-being Includes childhood development, primary, secondary, and higher education, and language and literacy skills	Education attainment[11] → increased health knowledge, health literacy and health-promoting behaviors, affecting factors such as nutrition, exercise, tobacco use, health, and disease management Educational attainment[11] → increased employment opportunities, affecting income work-related resources and benefits
Health-care access and quality	The connection between an individual's access to health care, its quality, and their health Includes access to primary health care, health-care insurance coverage and health literacy	Lack of health insurance[3] → less likelihood to have a primary care provider and less likelihood to afford health-care services and necessary medications Decreased health literacy[11] → reduced ability to make well-informed, positive health-related decisions, and difficulty with interpreting and acting on health-care decisions and management plans
Neighborhood and built environment	The connection between an individual's housing and environment and how these affect their health Includes housing quality, transportation, access to healthy and nutritious foods, water and air quality, and crime and violence	Neighborhood conditions and poor housing quality[3] → exposure to pest infestations and hazardous substances (mold, toxic chemicals, polluted water, lead paint), overcrowding and threats to public health and infectious disease spread Food insecurity[3] → malnutrition and reliance on nutrient-poor foods, causing or worsening disorders associated with nutritional deficits, obesity and metabolic consequences
Economic stability	The relationship between an individual's financial status and their health Includes employment, income, poverty status, food security, and housing stability	Lack of access to material goods and services due to low income[3] → poorer housing/living conditions and food insecurity (see "neighborhood and built environment"), inability to afford health-care services and treatment, inability to afford transportation for access to medical care
Social and community context	The relationship between where individuals grow, live, learn, work, and play and how these influence their health Includes social connection and cohesion, workplace conditions, incarceration, discrimination, and civic participation	High-risk working conditions can[11] → increased risk of injuries, exposure to hazardous chemicals, high noise levels, and inadequate ventilation Jobs with repetitive movements can[11] → musculoskeletal disorders Social connection[3] → increase in health behaviors and reduced emotional and psychological distress

central role of racism in all its forms, both in its historical context as well as in its present-day manifestations. This topic is discussed in detail in Articles # 3, 4, and 5.

Social Determinants of Health in Dermatology

The evidence of health and health-care disparities in dermatology is growing, in the areas of access to care, patient experiences, diagnosis, treatment, and dermatologic health outcomes. The underlying reasons for these disparities are broad and multifactorial, ranging from the SDoH, systemic and structural racism, knowledge gaps in skin of color dermatology, a lack of diverse and equitable representation in the dermatology workforce, a lack of research on dermatologic conditions disproportionately affecting minority populations, a lack of inclusivity of racial and ethnic minority patients in dermatology research, and the presence of unconscious/implicit bias among dermatology clinicians.[23,24] Extrapolating the influence of the SDoH from other factors that lead to disparities and health inequity is challenging because of the intertwined and interdependent nature of these factors. This review focuses on the influence of the SDoH health for patients with dermatologic disease. It is not comprehensive of every dermatologic disease that may be reported in the literature as being associated with some facet of the SDoH but rather focuses on areas that have more data.

Atopic dermatitis

The prevalence of atopic dermatitis (AD) is higher in Black children as compared with White children, and Black and Hispanic children also have more severe and persistent disease.[25–27] Although the relationship between SES and AD remains unclear, with a recent systematic review demonstrating inconsistent data,[28] it is clear that barriers to care for patients with low SES include decreased access to care providers and specialists[29] and difficulty affording over-the-counter treatments and prescription medications.[30] Black and Hispanic children have been shown to be more likely to have persistent AD[26] with more severe disease[27] because of decreased access to quality health care. The economic burden of AD is also well established and encompasses direct and indirect costs.[31,32] The cumulative effect of these challenges for AD patients of low SES is a decreased ability to control their disease, which could account for reports of higher disease severity in this population.[31]

Neighborhood and built environment factors contribute to further harm. Black, Hispanic, and indigenous communities are more frequently exposed to environmental hazards, pollutants, toxins, and other effects of poor housing,[33–35] all of which are associated with AD.[36] In one survey, AD severity was associated with Black/African American race, Hispanic ethnicity, lower household income, a home with a single mother, lower caregiver/parental educational level, worse maternal general health, lower household income, exposure to tobacco smoke and fair or poor maternal health.[36]

Highlighting the influence of structural racism in AD is the evidence that merely living in segregated communities (the modern day manifestation of historical redlining) predisposes Black/African American children to increased AD severity.[36] Historically, policies dictating highway placement and toxic waste sites targeted redlined census tracts.[34,37,38] As a result, redlining created areas with higher levels of hazardous air pollutants. Air quality and both indoor and outdoor pollutants have been shown to trigger and/or exacerbate AD in children.[39] One study in California revealed historically redlined census tracts as having significantly higher rates of emergency department visits due to asthma.[34]

Psoriasis

There is a dearth of research on the impacts of the SDoH in psoriasis. Lower educational level has been demonstrated to be associated with more severe disease and poorer control of psoriasis in adult patients.[40] Psoriasis is a disorder of systemic inflammation with evidence that obesity is a predisposing risk factor for both development of psoriasis and severity, particularly given its inherently inflammatory effect.[41,42] Obesity in the United States occurs at higher levels in individuals with lower incomes and lower educational levels.[43] Smoking has also been shown to be a risk a factor for psoriasis and can also negatively influence the benefit of certain systemic treatments.[44] Individuals with low SES are at higher risk of smoking behavior, thus putting them at increased risk of the harmful sequelae of smoking.[45,46]

Hidradenitis suppurativa

As with psoriasis, there is a lack of research on the direct relationship of the SDoH in hidradenitis suppurativa (HS). HS has been shown to be most prominent in Black/African American individuals as compared with any other race,[47–49] and one study showed that Hispanic patients have increased disease severity.[50] Patients in the United States with hidradenitis have been shown to be more likely to have low SES compared with patients without HS, although this study did not control for other factors such as tobacco use, obesity, and race[51]; however, the finding of lower

SES in HS patients was also seen in a study with Dutch patients.[52] Black and Hispanic patients HS have been shown to have lower levels of education and household incomes, which ultimately could affect access to care.[50] HS in turn is known to have significant economic impact for patients, including slower income growth, higher rates of unemployment, and higher overall indirect costs.[53] This adds complicating factors for HS patient who are at lower SES levels. Behavioral factors are well known to be associated with HS, including obesity and smoking. A meta-analysis revealed that HS patients are 4 times more likely to be obese as compared with the general population,[54] and patients with HS who are active smokers have a greater number of body sites affected that HS patients who do not smoke or have quit smoking.[55] As stated above, with obesity and smoking being more prevalent in lower SES populations, this makes the SDoH important considerations in HS patients.

For both psoriasis and HS, as well as other dermatologic disorders that may be connected to behaviors and lifestyle factors such as diet and tobacco use, the therapeutic benefit of diet modification, physical activity, weight loss, smoking cessation in these conditions may be dependent on a variety on SDoH categories, such as education, economic stability, health literacy, health-care access, neighborhood environment, and social and community context.

Melanoma

There are stark racial and ethnic disparities for melanoma. A comprehensive review of all the data that exists on this subject is beyond the scope of this article but we will highlight the most relevant data on the influences of SDoH on melanoma outcomes. Non-White patients with melanoma have worse survival rates as compared with White patients, and non-Hispanic Black patients with melanoma are diagnosed at later stages and disproportionately have the highest percentages of late-stage disease and highest rates of melanoma mortality despite the higher incidence of melanoma in White patients.[56–60] In regional and distant metastatic disease, the disparity is worsening in Hispanic patients and even when controlling for anatomic site, all racial and ethnic minorities present with more advanced disease and worse survival rates.[59–61] When stage is adjusted for, there is no difference in melanoma-specific mortality, providing evidence for the fact that the differences in melanoma mortality can be attributed in part to disparities in delayed diagnosis as well as delayed and/or disparate treatment of racial and ethnic minorities.[56]

Individuals of lower SES are diagnosed with more thicker melanoma tumors and, as a result, experience higher case-fatality rates.[62,63] This is in part due to challenges in access to care. Individuals with lower SES have decreased access to dermatologists, which leads to delays in diagnosis and treatment and thus contributes to worse survival rates.[62,64,65] Educational level has also been shown to be inversely related to melanoma tumor thickness at the time of diagnosis, such that those with a higher educational level present with thinner tumors as compared to those with a lower educational level.[66] Reasons for this include less perception of the risks of melanoma among individuals with lower SES, as well as less knowledge about the seriousness of melanoma and self-detection practices.[66] Physicians are also less likely to provide knowledge about melanoma risk factors, screening, and self-detection methods to patients who have less education.[66]

Insurance status also affects melanoma outcomes. Patients with Medicaid or Medicare coverage and uninsured patients have been shown to be less likely to see a dermatologist as compared with privately insured patients.[67] Patients with Medicaid insurance are more likely to have a delay of more than 6 weeks to surgery for definitive therapeutic excision, as compared with those with private insurance.[68] In a review by Cortez and colleagues,[69] it is reported that individuals with Medicaid insurance have been shown to have a higher incidence of thicker melanomas, more advanced staging, and ulcerated tumors at time of diagnosis, as compared with individuals with private insurance. This affects racial and ethnic minorities given that non-White individuals in the United States have disproportionately higher rates of Medicaid coverage.[70] Individuals who are uninsured are also more likely to present with thicker tumors, more advanced disease, and are less likely to receive certain treatments, worsening their survival outcomes.[71] Individuals living in rural areas are also more likely to experience delays in access to care including obtaining a biopsy of their melanomas and referral to dermatologists, compared with individuals living in urban environments.[72,73]

SUMMARY

Improving the health of all individuals, regardless of their personal circumstances and barriers to care, is a paramount to achieving health equity. A reduction in health disparities is the yardstick by which equity can be measured. The upstream structural determinants of health shape and influence the downstream SDoH, which significantly influence the health and well-being of individuals and communities. Dermatology is no exception, and a variety of dermatologic disorders have growing evidence of disparities that are connected to the SDoH, including AD, psoriasis, HS, and melanoma. Understanding and taking action to address the SDoH is critical to improving the health experiences and health outcomes of all patients, and this will be discussed in Part 2, along with SDoH clinical care points related to the point of care.

CLINICS CARE POINTS

- The social determinants of health impact dermatologic health and health outcomes for a variety of conditions, including atopic dermatitis, psoriasis, hidradenitis suppurativa and melanoma.

- Collecting information on how patients are experiencing the social determinants of health is a necessary and crucial step in providing patient-centered care and improving dermatologic health outcomes. This information can be gathered by electronic medical record systems, patient questionnaires, and/or specific questions asked in the clinical visit.

- From individual clinicians to large institutions, health care delivery that is informed by each patient's social determinants of health data may have significant positive impacts for the patient's healthcare experience, disease activity, morbidity and mortality.

DISCLOSURE

There are no conflicts of interest or funding sources to disclose for Sacharitha Bowers. There are no conflicts of interest for Aileen Chang, however, Dr. Chang is supported by the Dermatology Foundation Public Health Career Development Award.

REFERENCES

1. Health Equity | CDC. 2022. Available at: https://www.cdc.gov/chronicdisease/healthequity/index.htm. Accessed May 22, 2022.
2. Social determinants of health. Available at: https://www.who.int/health-topics/social-determinants-of-health. Accessed April 29, 2022.
3. Social Determinants of Health - Healthy People 2030 | health.gov. Available at: https://health.gov/healthy people/priority-areas/social-determinants-health. Accessed May 22, 2022.
4. Daniel H, Bornstein SS, Kane GC. Addressing social determinants to improve patient care and promote health equity: an american college of physicians position paper. Ann Intern Med 2018;168(8):577–8.
5. Hood CM, Gennuso KP, Swain GR, et al. County health rankings: relationships between determinant factors and health outcomes. Am J Prev Med 2016;50(2):129–35.
6. U.S. Health Care from a Global Perspective, 2019: Higher Spending, Worse Outcomes? doi:10.26099/7avy-fc29
7. Taylor LA, Tan AX, Coyle CE, et al. Leveraging the Social Determinants of Health: What Works? PLoS One 2016;11(8):e0160217.
8. Rosen G. A history of public health. Baltimore: Johns Hopkins Univ. Press; 1993.
9. Braveman P, Gottlieb L. The social determinants of health: it's time to consider the causes of the causes. Public Health Rep 2014;129(Suppl 2):19–31.
10. Galea S, Tracy M, Hoggatt KJ, et al. Estimated deaths attributable to social factors in the United States. Am J Public Health 2011;101(8):1456–65.
11. Braveman P, Egerter S, Williams DR. The social determinants of health: coming of age. Annu Rev Public Health 2011;32(1):381–98.
12. Bharmal N, Derose KP, Felician M, et al. Understanding the Upstream Social Determinants of Health. Working Paper - RAND Social Determinants of Health Interest Group 2015.
13. About Social Determinants of Health (SDOH). 2021. Available at: https://www.cdc.gov/socialdeterminants/about.html. Accessed June 12, 2022.
14. A Conceptual Framework for Action on the Social Determinants of Health. Available at: https://www.who.int/publications-detail-redirect/9789241500852. Accessed May 21, 2022.
15. The BARHII Framework. BARHII. Available at: https://www.barhii.org/barhii-framework. Accessed April 26, 2022.
16. Link BG, Phelan J. Social Conditions As Fundamental Causes of Disease. J Health Soc Behav 1995;80–94. https://doi.org/10.2307/2626958.
17. Socioeconomic Status. Available at: https://www.apa.org/topics/socioeconomic-status. Accessed May 29, 2022.
18. Bureau UC. Inequalities Persist Despite Decline in Poverty For All Major Race and Hispanic Origin Groups. Census.gov. Available at: https://www.census.gov/library/stories/2020/09/poverty-rates-for-blacks-and-hispanics-reached-historic-lows-in-2019.html. Accessed May 29, 2022.
19. Lidsky TI, Schneider JS. Lead neurotoxicity in children: basic mechanisms and clinical correlates. Brain 2003;126(Pt 1):5–19.
20. Afeiche M, Peterson KE, Sánchez BN, et al. Windows of lead exposure sensitivity, attained height,

and body mass index at 48 months. J Pediatr 2012; 160(6):1044–9.

21. Brown P. Race, class, and environmental health: a review and systematization of the literature. Environ Res 1995;69(1):15–30.

22. Lanphear BP, Kahn RS, Berger O, et al. Contribution of residential exposures to asthma in us children and adolescents. Pediatrics 2001;107(6):E98.

23. Hooper J, Shao K, Feng H. Racial/Ethnic Health Disparities in Dermatology in the United States Part 1: Overview of Contributing Factors and Management Strategies. J Am Acad Dermatol 2022;0(0). https://doi.org/10.1016/j.jaad.2021.12.061.

24. Williams J, Amerson EH, Chang AY. How dermatologists can address the structural and social determinants of health—from awareness to action. JAMA Dermatol 2022. https://doi.org/10.1001/jamadermatol.2021.5925.

25. Brunner PM, Guttman-Yassky E. Racial differences in atopic dermatitis. Ann Allergy Asthma Immunol 2019;122(5):449–55.

26. Kim Y, Blomberg M, Rifas-Shiman SL, et al. Racial/ethnic differences in incidence and persistence of childhood atopic dermatitis. J Invest Dermatol 2019;139(4):827–34.

27. Silverberg JI, Simpson EL. Associations of childhood eczema severity: a US population based study. Dermatitis 2014;25(3):107–14. https://doi.org/10.1097/DER.0000000000000034.

28. Bajwa H, Baghchechi M, Mujahid M, et al. Mixed evidence on the relationship between socioeconomic position and atopic dermatitis: a systematic review. J Am Acad Dermatol 2022;86(2):399–405.

29. Alghothani L, Jacks SK, Vander Horst A, et al. Disparities in access to dermatologic care according to insurance type. Arch Dermatol 2012;148(8):956–7.

30. Silverberg JI. Health care utilization, patient costs, and access to care in US adults with eczema: a population-based study. JAMA Dermatol 2015;151(7):743–52.

31. Chung J, Simpson EL. The socioeconomics of atopic dermatitis. Ann Allergy Asthma Immunol 2019;122(4):360–6.

32. Murota H, Katayama I. Impairment of productivity in the workplace/classroom in japanese patients with atopic dermatitis. In: Katayama I, Murota H, Satoh T, editors. Evolution of atopic dermatitis in the 21st century. Springer; 2018. p. 321–8. https://doi.org/10.1007/978-981-10-5541-6_25.

33. Bailey ZD, Feldman JM, Bassett MT. How structural racism works — racist policies as a root cause of U.S. Racial health inequities. N Engl J Med 2021; 384(8):768–73.

34. Nardone A, Casey JA, Morello-Frosch R, et al. Associations between historical residential redlining and current age-adjusted rates of emergency

department visits due to asthma across eight cities in California: an ecological study. Lancet Planet Health 2020;4(1):e24–31.

35. Rosenbaum E. Racial/ethnic differences in asthma prevalence: the role of housing and neighborhood environments. J Health Soc Behav 2008;49(2): 131–45.

36. Tackett KJ, Jenkins F, Morrell DS, et al. Structural racism and its influence on the severity of atopic dermatitis in African American children. Pediatr Dermatol 2020;37(1):142–6.

37. Rothstein R. The color of law. New York: Liveright Publishing Corporation; 2018.

38. Whittemore AH. The experience of racial and ethnic minorities with zoning in the United States. J Plann Lit 2017;32(1):16–27.

39. Kantor R, Silverberg JI. Environmental risk factors and their role in the management of atopic dermatitis. Expert Rev Clin Immunol 2017;13(1): 15–26.

40. Kimball Ab, Augustin M, Gordon Kb, et al. Correlation of psoriasis activity with socioeconomic status: cross-sectional analysis of patients enrolled in the Psoriasis Longitudinal Assessment and Registry (PSOLAR). Br J Dermatol 2018;179(4):984–6.

41. Jensen P, Skov L. Psoriasis and Obesity. DRM 2016; 232(6):633–9.

42. Xu C, Ji J, Su T, et al. The association of psoriasis and obesity: focusing on IL-17A-related immunological mechanisms. Int J Dermatol Venereol 2021;4(2): 116–21.

43. Christopher G, Fleming D, Harris RT, et al. The State of Obesity: 2021: Better Policies for a Healthier America. Trust for America's Health 18th Annual Report. https://www.tfah.org/report-details/state-of-obesity-2021/.

44. Zhou H, Wu R, Kong Y, et al. Impact of smoking on psoriasis risk and treatment efficacy: a meta-analysis. J Int Med Res 2020;48(10). 0300060520964024.

45. Garrett BE, Dube SR, Babb S, et al. Addressing the social determinants of health to reduce tobacco-related disparities. Nicotine Tob Res 2015;17(8): 892–7.

46. Upson D. Social determinants of cigarette smoking. Tob Epidemic 2015;42:181–98.

47. Garg A, Kirby JS, Lavian J, et al. Sex- and age-adjusted population analysis of prevalence estimates for hidradenitis suppurativa in the United States. JAMA Dermatol 2017;153(8):760–4.

48. McMillan K. Hidradenitis suppurativa: number of diagnosed patients, demographic characteristics, and treatment patterns in the United States. Am J Epidemiol 2014;179(12):1477–83.

49. Sachdeva M, Shah M, Alavi A. Race-specific prevalence of hidradenitis suppurativa. J Cutan Med Surg 2021;25(2):177–87.

50. Kilgour JM, Li S, Sarin KY. Hidradenitis suppurativa in patients of color is associated with increased disease severity and healthcare utilization: a retrospective analysis of 2 U.S. cohorts. JAAD Int 2021;3: 42–52.

51. Wertenteil S, Strunk A, Garg A. Association of low socioeconomic status with hidradenitis suppurativa in the United States. JAMA Dermatol 2018;154(9): 1086–8.

52. Deckers IE, Janse IC, van der Zee HH, et al. Hidradenitis suppurativa (HS) is associated with low socioeconomic status (SES): a cross-sectional reference study. J Am Acad Dermatol 2016;75(4): 755–9.e1.

53. Tzellos T, Yang H, Mu F, et al. Impact of hidradenitis suppurativa on work loss, indirect costs and income. Br J Dermatol 2019;181(1):147–54.

54. Choi F, Lehmer L, Ekelem C, et al. Dietary and metabolic factors in the pathogenesis of hidradenitis suppurativa: a systematic review. Int J Dermatol 2020; 59(2):143–53.

55. Bukvić Mokos Z, Miše J, Balić A, et al. Understanding the relationship between smoking and hidradenitis suppurativa. Acta Dermatovenerol Croat 2020; 28(1):9–13.

56. Brady J, Kashlan R, Ruterbusch J, et al. Racial disparities in patients with melanoma: a multivariate survival analysis. Clin Cosmet Investig Dermatol 2021;14:547–50.

57. Wang Y, Zhao Y, Ma S. Racial differences in six major subtypes of melanoma: descriptive epidemiology. BMC Cancer 2016;16(1):691.

58. Dawes SM, Tsai S, Gittleman H, et al. Racial disparities in melanoma survival. J Am Acad Dermatol 2016;75(5):983–91.

59. Cormier JN, Xing Y, Ding M, et al. Ethnic differences among patients with cutaneous melanoma. Arch Intern Med 2006;166(17):1907–14.

60. Qian Y, Johannet P, Sawyers A, et al. The ongoing racial disparities in melanoma: An analysis of the Surveillance, Epidemiology, and End Results database (1975-2016). J Am Acad Dermatol 2021; 84(6):1585–93.

61. Stubblefield J, Kelly B. Melanoma in non-caucasian populations. Surg Clin North Am 2014;94(5): 1115–1126, ix.

62. Ortiz CAR, Goodwin JS, Freeman JL. The effect of socioeconomic factors on incidence, stage at diagnosis and survival of cutaneous melanoma. Med Sci Monit 2005;11(5):RA163–72.

63. Youl PH, Baade PD, Parekh S, et al. Association between melanoma thickness, clinical skin examination and socioeconomic status: results of a large population-based study. Int J Cancer 2011;128(9): 2158–65.

64. Zell JA, Cinar P, Mobasher M, et al. Survival for patients with invasive cutaneous melanoma among ethnic groups: the effects of socioeconomic status and treatment. J Clin Oncol 2008;26(1):66–75.

65. Mavor ME, Richardson H, Miao Q, et al. Disparities in diagnosis of advanced melanoma: a population-based cohort study. Can Med Assoc Open Access J 2018;6(4):E502–12.

66. Pollitt RA, Swetter SM, Johnson TM, et al. Examining the pathways linking lower socioeconomic status and advanced melanoma. Cancer 2012;118(16): 4004–13.

67. Tripathi R, Knusel KD, Ezaldein HH, et al. Association of Demographic and Socioeconomic Characteristics With Differences in Use of Outpatient Dermatology Services in the United States. JAMA Dermatol 2018;154(11):1286–91.

68. Adamson AS, Zhou L, Baggett CD, et al. Association of Delays in Surgery for Melanoma With Insurance Type. JAMA Dermatol 2017;153(11):1106–13.

69. Cortez JL, Vasquez J, Wei ML. The impact of demographics, socioeconomics, and health care access on melanoma outcomes. J Am Acad Dermatol 2021;84(6):1677–83.

70. Distribution of the Nonelderly with Medicaid by Race/Ethnicity. KFF. 2020. Available at: https://www.kff.org/medicaid/state-indicator/medicaid-distribution-nonelderly-by-raceethnicity/. Accessed June 8, 2022.

71. Amini A, Rusthoven CG, Waxweiler TV, et al. Association of health insurance with outcomes in adults ages 18 to 64 years with melanoma in the United States. J Am Acad Dermatol 2016;74(2):309–16.

72. Strömberg U, Peterson S, Holmberg E, et al. Cutaneous malignant melanoma show geographic and socioeconomic disparities in stage at diagnosis and excess mortality. Acta Oncol 2016;55(8): 993–1000.

73. Feng H, Berk-Krauss J, Feng PW, et al. Comparison of dermatologist density between urban and rural counties in the United States. JAMA Dermatol 2018;154(11):1265–71.

The Social Determinants of Health and Their Impact on Dermatologic Health, Part 2
Taking Action to Address the Social Determinants of Health

Aileen Y. Chang, MD[a],*, Sacharitha Bowers, MD[b]

KEYWORDS

- Social determinants of health • Access to care • Health-related social needs

KEY POINTS

- The social determinants of health (SDoH) are nonmedical factors that greatly influence the health and well-being of individuals, across every discipline in medicine, including dermatology.
- Improving dermatology health outcomes requires an understanding of the SDoH and how they impact dermatologic health and lead to disparities in patients with dermatologic disorders.
- Identifying, accommodating, and assisting with health-related social needs at the point of care is an evidence-based and actionable strategy that dermatologists can use to address the impact of the SDoH in the health care setting.
- Outside the clinic walls, alignment with communities and engaging in advocacy work can further help to mitigate the impact of the SDoH as well as address their upstream causes.

INTRODUCTION

In part due to disparities highlighted by the COVID-19 pandemic, there has been a renewed emphasis on health equity—the ability of every individual to attain their "full health potential" and not be "disadvantaged from achieving this potential due to social position or other socially determined circumstances."[1] Health equity can be measured by the state of health disparities. Knowledge on the factors that impact the health and well-being of individuals and communities, including the contributors to health disparities and health equity, has expanded due to a deeper understanding of the factors outside an individual's control—namely, the social determinants of health (SDoH). The SDoH, defined as *the conditions in which people are born, grow, live, learn, work, play, and age*,[2,3] contribute to health outcomes and health disparities to a far greater degree than access to health care alone.[4,5]

The SDoH have been shown to contribute to widening dermatologic health disparities. Dermatologists must become aware of how the SDoH affect the health of our patients with cutaneous conditions so they can be well-equipped to meet their patients' needs and decrease dermatologic disparities. Part 1 of this 2-part series reviewed

Disclosure: The authors have no commercial or financial conflicts of interest to disclose. Dr A.Y. Chang is supported by a Dermatology Foundation Public Health Career Development Award.
[a] Department of Dermatology, University of California San Francisco, Zuckerberg San Francisco General Hospital, 995 Potrero Avenue, Building 90, Ward 92, San Francisco, CA 94110, USA; [b] Division of Dermatology, Department of Internal Medicine, Southern Illinois University School of Medicine, 751 North Rutledge Suite 2300, Springfield, IL 62702, USA
* Corresponding author.
E-mail address: aileen.chang@ucsf.edu

Dermatol Clin 41 (2023) 317–324
https://doi.org/10.1016/j.det.2022.10.010
0733-8635/23/© 2022 Elsevier Inc. All rights reserved.

the nature of the SDoH, how they can impact overall health, and their implications in dermatologic disease and health outcomes. Part 2 aims to provide dermatology practitioners and trainees guidance on interventions that can be taken to modify the harmful impacts of the SDoH.

TAKING ACTION: HEALTH-RELATED SOCIAL NEEDS
Defining Health-Related Social Needs

Although the term "social determinants of health" is colloquially used to convey a need for a particular resource or support, it is itself a neutral term (eg, housing, food access, transportation). In contrast, terms such as "social needs," "social risks,[6]" and "health-related social needs (HRSNs)" are more appropriate to use when communicating an individual's lack of a particular resource or support. HRSN is one of the specific terms used to describe a social need that cannot be treated by medical care (eg, unstable housing, food insecurity, and transportation difficulties)[7,8] and if left unmet, may increase an individual's risk of developing a health condition, limit an individual's ability to manage a health condition, and/or increase health care utilization and costs that might otherwise have been avoided.

Commonly Reported Social Needs in Clinical Settings

The most common social needs reported by patients in clinical settings are related to housing, food, child care, and financial strain.[9] Housing-related needs include housing instability and being unhoused as well as low-quality housing and limited space in the home.[9] Food-related needs include eating less, skipping meals, and not having enough food to feed one's family.[9] Child care-related needs include the need to find affordable and quality child care.[9] Financial strain includes not having enough money for unexpected expenses or health care as well as general employment and income concerns.[9]

Health-Related Social Needs and Increased Health Care Utilization

Health systems, payers, and public health organizations have taken a growing interest in identifying and addressing unmet HRSNs, as patients who are high-utilizers of health care often have one or more unmet HRSNs.[8,10–12] As compared with having one HRSN, having multiple, concurrent HRSNs was strongly associated with an increased risk of two or more emergency department (ED) visits,[8] having two or more HRSNs was positively

associated with ED visits and negatively associated with wellness visits,[10] and patients with the most number of social risks had the highest utilization of care, despite being younger and having the fewest medical comorbidities.[11] In addition to the large body of literature focused on the impact of interventions for social and economic needs on process and social outcomes,[13] there is growing data to support social needs interventions as a means to reducing health care utilization in patients with complex medical and social needs[14,15] as well as high-utilizing patients in safety-net settings[16] and integrated health systems.[17]

Health-Related Social Needs Among Specific Populations

HRSNs and challenges related to SDoH are not randomly distributed across a population. As SDoH are heavily influenced by society's social and economic policies, individuals from the same neighborhood or community often have similar HRSNs. These social needs and the barriers to addressing them are interconnected and have subsequent impact on the health of individuals and their communities. As such, there is expanding effort to integrate individual-level SDoH data with community-level SDoH data[18] to inform community-based interventions in neighborhoods with a high burden of HRSNs.

Identifying specific population subgroups at increased risk for having one or more HRSNs has important implications for addressing equity when designing and implementing individual-level and community-level interventions to address HRSNs. National surveillance data suggest that individuals identifying as a racial and ethnic minority are at increased risk for housing instability and food insecurity.[19–21] However, studies to-date report an inconsistent association between race/ethnicity and social needs, which may reflect differences in study sample and measurement of social needs.[9]

Health-Related Social Needs Screening in Clinical Care

Screening for HRSNs in the health care setting has been championed by many organizations, including the American Medical Association, the National Academies of Sciences, Engineering, and Medicine, and the Centers for Medicare and Medicaid Services.[7,22,23] Studies evaluating patient and clinician acceptability of social needs screening in clinic have highlighted important considerations for implementation of social needs screening in clinical care.

Patient Perspectives on Screening

Multiple studies evaluating patient perspectives on social needs screening have been conducted in adult and pediatric primary care and ED settings. In one study of 969 adult patients and adult caregivers of pediatric patients recruited from six primary care clinics and four EDs across nine states, higher perceived screening appropriateness was associated with previously having been asked about social needs in a health care setting, trust in clinicians, and having been recruited for the study from a primary care clinic rather than the ED; lower appropriateness was associated with previous experience of health care discrimination.[24] In another study of 1161 adult participants across seven clinical sites within an integrated health system in California, most respondents agreed that social needs impact health (69%), their health system should ask about social needs (85%), and help address social needs (88%).[25]

Patient participants have also expressed concerns related to privacy and confidentiality.[26] These concerns can be influenced by prior experiences in the health care system with bias and discrimination. Patients also express concern with their screening information being shared outside of their health care team or other patients becoming aware of their screening responses. Yet, patients also acknowledge that collection and documentation of social needs is often necessary to be able to offer assistance.[26]

Clinician Perspectives on Screening

Studies evaluating clinician perspectives on social needs screening in the health care setting have occurred within academic medical centers, large integrated health systems, and safety-net clinics.[27–31] Most of the clinicians agree that SDoH and social need information is important to clinical care.[27–29,31] However, barriers to incorporating social needs screening include the lack of time to identify and address social needs,[28,30,31] lack of resources to identify, address, and/or follow-up on social needs,[27–29,31] lack of support staff to ask,[29] lack of training to respond to identified needs.[27–29,31] Other concerns raised by clinicians include unintended consequences of screening,[28] patients' fears and concerns related to confidentiality and privacy,[28,30] promoting feelings of stigma or shame through screening.[28] Being able to address social needs has also been identified as a strategy for prevention of burnout; being able to address patients' social needs may lead to greater job satisfaction.[30]

One study from an academic medical center in Florida evaluated differences in perspective based on the faculty member belonging to a racial ethnic minority group and whether primary care provider (PCP) or specialist.[27] Within minority faculty and PCPs, the second most common concern about collecting SDoH information was liability related to not addressing an identified social risk that leads to an adverse outcome, as compared with not knowing how to use SDoH information for nonminority faculty and specialists.[27] Furthermore, belonging to a racial ethnic minority group was the only factor associated with believing that the benefits of collecting SDoH data outweigh the risks.[27] This suggests that the racial/ethnic composition of clinicians may impact engagement and support for collecting SDoH data,[27] potentially as a result of lived experiences.[32]

FRAMEWORK FOR DERMATOLOGISTS

Dermatology patients are faced with SDoH challenges, and dermatologists often wonder what they can do to help their patients. The National Academies of Sciences, Engineering, and Medicine report, *Integrating Social Care into the Delivery of Health Care*, defined five types of social care activities that health care providers can engage in (the "5 As")[22]:

- *Awareness:* Identify the social risks and assets of defined patients and population
- *Adjustment:* Alter clinical care to accommodate identified social barriers
- *Assistance:* Reduce social risk by providing assistance in connecting patients with relevant social care resources
- *Alignment:* Understand existing social care assets in the community, organize them to facilitate synergies, and invest in and deploy them to positively affect health outcomes.
- *Advocacy:* Work with partner social care organizations to promote policies that facilitate the creation and redeployment of assets or resources to address health and social needs.

Dermatologists can use this framework to mobilize as individuals and collectively to identify and address HRSNs affecting their patients.[33] As put forth in this framework,[22] the first "3 As" of awareness, assistance, and adjustment are most applicable to dermatologists in clinic. **Table 1** details how dermatologists can ask, adjust, and assist with their patients experiencing SDoH challenges. Asking about SDoH (awareness) is a fundamental activity that must precede any other action. It is also vital to understand what resources are

Table 1
Identifying and addressing social needs in dermatology at point of care

Identifying and Addressing SDoH Challenges in Dermatology Clinic			
SDoH	Ask	Adjust	Assist
Housing	Open-ended questions that include rationale are ideal for asking about housing status, which is a sensitive topic: • "I'd like to ask you some questions about your housing situation so I can better understand what treatments may be more feasible. What is your housing situation today?" • "Sometimes people who cannot bathe once weekly experience an itchy rash similar to yours. When was the last time you were able to take a bath or shower?" Direct questions for housing • "What is your housing situation today?" • "Where do you stay?"	Lack of privacy and/or access to clean water → Consider choosing a systemic therapy over a topical therapy Lack of refrigeration access → See if biologic therapy can be ordered to and stored at your clinic's pharmacy or nearby pharmacy. Patient can pick up from the pharmacy and come to clinic for the injection See transportation section for more adjustment activities	Crucial to understand what resources are available within health care organization and local community before asking about social needs Refer to appropriate resources in health care organization or community Refer to patient navigator or social worker in your health care organization or community
Transportation	Open-ended questions are ideal to begin the conversation and then ask more directed questions as needed: • "I look forward to continuing to work with you on this. I wonder, what challenges might you have getting to our clinic in the future?" Direct questions for transportation: • "Do you think lack of reliable transportation will keep you from getting to our clinic or getting your medications?"	Difficulty getting to clinic, Unreliable phone access—> Create safe, low barrier environment to access care: • Drop-in, evening, and/or weekend hours • Make next appointment in clinic before leaving • Telemedicine visits	Keep a clinic supply of bus tokens or fare cards, cab vouchers Some health care systems subsidize transportation Refer to appropriate resources in health care organization or community Refer to patient navigator or social worker in your health care organization or community
Health insurance	*Direct, contextualized questions for health insurance:* "In order to make sure we have a good long-	If paying out-of-pocket for meds, options to reduce cost include: • $4 generic meds at Target, Walmart	Refer to eligibility office in health care organization or community. If possible, patient

(continued on next page)

Table 1 *(continued)*			
Identifying and Addressing SDoH Challenges in Dermatology Clinic			
SDoH	**Ask**	**Adjust**	**Assist**
	term plan for your psoriasis, we need to know your health insurance plan. If you don't have health insurance, we will make sure an eligibility staff member meets with you."	• GoodRx to view prices at local pharmacies and obtain coupons • Costco Pharmacy: search price online (members get discounted pricing) • Amazon Pharmacy: search price online (Prime members may have additional discounts)	should make contact while in clinic, especially if patient has limited English proficiency and clinic staff speak the patient's preferred language.
Language, health literacy	Sometimes it is evident that an interpreter is needed OR the dermatologist has already been made aware by clinic staff. Even if you are in a clinical setting with many patients with limited English proficiency, do not assume the patient's preferred language. Best to ask the patient. "Before we start talking, I want to ask you about what language we should use today. What language do you prefer to speak?. . . I don't speak [language], so let's ask an interpreter to help us." "What language do you speak?"	Incorporate best practices for using a medical interpreter (additional tips in Table 1 of this citation[36]) - Use first-person statements ("I" statements); avoid "tell the patient", "ask her" -Speak in short thought groups, group together short sentences. -Prioritize key points to three or fewer Use "teach-back" to ensure patient understood key information. Unfortunately, even with the use of a qualified interpreter, effective communication can still be a challenge when there is language discordance between the patient and clinician	Use of qualified interpreters is associated with improved clinical care[37] and federally mandated in the United States for health care organizations receiving federal funding.[38,39]

available within a health care organization and the local community—and how these resources can be accessed—before asking patients about their social needs.

In addition to the awareness, adjustment, and assistance activities discussed in **Table 1**, dermatologists as individuals and an organized body can engage in alignment and advocacy activities. Community engagement and partnership will enable dermatologists to understand directly from local communities affected by unmet social needs what their prioritized needs are and how dermatologists can be effective in supporting, and investing in, the communities they serve. These alignment activities will also help inform advocacy activities, wherein dermatologists can be engaged with policy change at the local, state, and national level that directly impacts the social and economic policies that influence SDoH.[33]

CLINICS CARE POINTS

At the point of care, dermatologists can use the first "3 As" of the National Academies of Sciences, Engineering, and Medicine (NASEM) framework to identify and address social needs related to their patients:

- *Awareness:* Identify the social risks and assets of defined patients and population
- *Adjustment:* Alter clinical care to accommodate identified social barriers
- *Assistance:* Reduce social risk by providing assistance in connecting patients with relevant social care resources

Table 1 provides details for each of these actions, organized by common SDoH challenges in dermatology. Limited English proficiency is included because limited English proficiency in a primarily English-speaking country is associated with low health literacy[34,35]—an important SDoH.

SUMMARY

Dermatology practitioners should be well-equipped to better address the health needs of all their patients, regardless of their personal circumstances and barriers to care. Beyond gaining the knowledge about the SDoH and how they contribute to health disparities, dermatology clinicians can engage in individual behaviors at the point of care to address their patients' social needs. They can also participate and organize in alignment and advocacy efforts to target change upstream that impacts health. Advancing equity is possible, but only with awareness followed by intentional action, and this review aims to be a step in that direction.

REFERENCES

1. Health Equity | CDC. 2022. Available at: https://www.cdc.gov/chronicdisease/healthequity/index.htm. Accessed May 22, 2022.
2. Social determinants of health. Available at: https://www.who.int/health-topics/social-determinants-of-health. Accessed April 29, 2022.
3. Social Determinants of Health - Healthy People 2030 | health.gov. Available at: https://health.gov/healthypeople/priority-areas/social-determinants-health. Accessed May 22, 2022.
4. Daniel H, Bornstein SS, Kane GC. Addressing Social Determinants to Improve Patient Care and Promote Health Equity: An American College of Physicians Position Paper. Ann Intern Med 2018;168(8):577–8. https://doi.org/10.7326/M17-2441.
5. Hood CM, Gennuso KP, Swain GR, et al. County Health Rankings: Relationships Between Determinant Factors and Health Outcomes. Am J Prev Med 2016;50(2):129–35. https://doi.org/10.1016/j.amepre.2015.08.024.
6. Alderwick H, Gottlieb LM. Meanings and Misunderstandings: A Social Determinants of Health Lexicon for Health Care Systems. Milbank Q 2019;97(2):407–19. https://doi.org/10.1111/1468-0009.12390.
7. Centers for Medicare and Medicaid Services. Accountable Health Communities Model. Available at: https://innovation.cms.gov/innovation-models/ahcm. Accessed April 19, 2022.
8. Holcomb J, Highfield L, Ferguson GM, et al. Association of Social Needs and Healthcare Utilization Among Medicare and Medicaid Beneficiaries in the Accountable Health Communities Model. J GEN INTERN MED 2022. https://doi.org/10.1007/s11606-022-07403-w.
9. Kreuter MW, Thompson T, McQueen A, et al. Addressing Social Needs in Health Care Settings: Evidence, Challenges, and Opportunities for Public Health. Annu Rev Public Health 2021;42:329–44. https://doi.org/10.1146/annurev-publhealth-090419-102204.
10. McQueen A, Li L, Herrick CJ, et al. Social Needs, Chronic Conditions, and Health Care Utilization among Medicaid Beneficiaries. Popul Health Manag 2021;24(6):681–90. https://doi.org/10.1089/pop.2021.0065.
11. Rogers A, Hu YR, Schickedanz A, et al. Understanding High-Utilizing Patients Based on Social Risk Profiles: a Latent Class Analysis Within an Integrated Health System. J Gen Intern Med 2020;35(7):2214–6. https://doi.org/10.1007/s11606-019-05510-9.
12. Blalock DV, Maciejewski ML, Zulman DM, et al. Subgroups of High-Risk Veterans Affairs Patients Based on Social Determinants of Health Predict Risk of Future Hospitalization. Med Care 2021;59(5):410–7. https://doi.org/10.1097/MLR.0000000000001526.
13. Gottlieb LM, Wing H, Adler NE. A Systematic Review of Interventions on Patients' Social and Economic Needs. Am J Prev Med 2017;53(5):719–29. https://doi.org/10.1016/j.amepre.2017.05.011.
14. Berkowitz SA, Terranova J, Hill C, et al. Meal Delivery Programs Reduce The Use Of Costly Health Care In Dually Eligible Medicare And Medicaid Beneficiaries. Health Aff (Millwood) 2018;37(4):535–42. https://doi.org/10.1377/hlthaff.2017.0999.
15. Baxter AJ, Tweed EJ, Katikireddi SV, et al. Effects of Housing First approaches on health and well-being of adults who are homeless or at risk of homelessness: systematic review and meta-analysis of

randomised controlled trials. J Epidemiol Community Health 2019;73(5):379–87. https://doi.org/10.1136/jech-2018-210981.

16. Lim S, Singh TP, Hall G, et al. Impact of a New York City Supportive Housing Program on Housing Stability and Preventable Health Care among Homeless Families. Health Serv Res 2018;53(5):3437–54. https://doi.org/10.1111/1475-6773.12849.

17. Schickedanz A, Sharp A, Hu YR, et al. Impact of Social Needs Navigation on Utilization Among High Utilizers in a Large Integrated Health System: a Quasi-experimental Study. J GEN INTERN MED 2019;34(11):2382–9. https://doi.org/10.1007/s11606-019-05123-2.

18. Hatef E, Ma X, Rouhizadeh M, et al. Assessing the Impact of Social Needs and Social Determinants of Health on Health Care Utilization: Using Patient- and Community-Level Data. Popul Health Manag 2021;24(2):222–30. https://doi.org/10.1089/pop.2020.0043.

19. US Department of Health and Human Services, Office of Disease Prevention and Health Promotion. Housing Instability. Healthy People. 2020. https://www.healthypeople.gov/2020/topics-objectives/topic/social-determinants-health/interventions-resources/housing-instability.

20. US Department of Health and Human Services, Office of Disease Prevention and Health Promotion. Food Insecurity Healthy People 2020. Available at: https://www.healthypeople.gov/2020/topics-objectives/topic/social-determinants-health/interventions-resources/food-insecurity.

21. US Department of Agriculture Economic Research Service. Food security and nutrition assistance. Economic Research Service. 2020. Available at: https://www.ers.usda.gov/data-products/ag-and-food-statistics-charting-the-essentials/food-security-and-nutrition-assistance/.

22. National Academies of Sciences, Engineering, and Medicine. Integrating Social Care into the Delivery of Health Care: Moving Upstream to Improve the Nation's Health. Natl Academies Press 2019. Available at: nationalacademies.org/SocialCare.

23. American Medical Association. H-160.896 Expanding Access to Screening Tools for Social Determ | AMA. Available at: https://policysearch.ama-assn.org/policyfinder/detail/Social%20determinants%20?uri=%2FAMADoc%2FHOD.xml-H-160.896.xml. Accessed May 2, 2022.

24. De Marchis EH, Hessler D, Fichtenberg C, et al. Part I: A Quantitative Study of Social Risk Screening Acceptability in Patients and Caregivers. Am J Prev Med 2019;57(6):S25–37. https://doi.org/10.1016/j.amepre.2019.07.010.

25. Rogers AJ, Hamity C, Sharp AL, et al. Patients' Attitudes and Perceptions Regarding Social Needs Screening and Navigation: Multi-site Survey in a Large Integrated Health System. J Gen Intern Med 2020;35(5):1389–95. https://doi.org/10.1007/s11606-019-05588-1.

26. Byhoff E, Marchis EHD, Hessler D, et al. Part II: A Qualitative Study of Social Risk Screening Acceptability in Patients and Caregivers. Am J Prev Med 2019;57(6):S38–46. https://doi.org/10.1016/j.amepre.2019.07.016.

27. Palacio A, Seo D, Medina H, et al. Provider Perspectives on the Collection of Social Determinants of Health. Popul Health Manag 2018;21(6):501–8. https://doi.org/10.1089/pop.2017.0166.

28. Sokol RL, Ammer J, Stein SF, et al. Provider Perspectives on Screening for Social Determinants of Health in Pediatric Settings: A Qualitative Study. J Pediatr Health Care 2021;35(6):577–86. https://doi.org/10.1016/j.pedhc.2021.08.004.

29. Kostelanetz S, Pettapiece-Phillips M, Weems J, et al. Health Care Professionals' Perspectives on Universal Screening of Social Determinants of Health: A Mixed-Methods Study. Popul Health Manag 2021. https://doi.org/10.1089/pop.2021.0176.

30. Nehme E, Castedo de Martell S, Matthews H, et al. Experiences and Perspectives on Adopting New Practices for Social Needs-targeted Care in Safety-net Settings: A Qualitative Case Series Study. J Prim Care Community Health 2021;12. https://doi.org/10.1177/21501327211017784. 21501327211017784.

31. Schickedanz A, Hamity C, Rogers A, et al. Clinician Experiences and Attitudes Regarding Screening for Social Determinants of Health in a Large Integrated Health System. Med Care 2019;57(Suppl 6 Suppl 2):S197–201. https://doi.org/10.1097/MLR.0000000000001051.

32. Palacio A, Tamariz L. Provider Perspectives When Integrating Social Determinants of Health in Response to Schickedanz A, Hamity C, Rogers A, et al, Clinician Experiences and Attitudes Regarding Screening for Social Determinants of Health in a Large Integrated Health System. Med Care 2020;58(2):192. https://doi.org/10.1097/MLR.0000000000001231.

33. Williams J, Amerson EH, Chang AY. How Dermatologists Can Address the Structural and Social Determinants of Health—From Awareness to Action. JAMA Dermatol 2022. https://doi.org/10.1001/jamadermatol.2021.5925.

34. Wilson E, Chen AHM, Grumbach K, et al. Effects of limited English proficiency and physician language on health care comprehension. J Gen Intern Med 2005;20(9):800–6. https://doi.org/10.1111/j.1525-1497.2005.0174.x.

35. Leyva M, Sharif I, Ozuah PO. Health literacy among Spanish-speaking Latino parents with limited English proficiency. Ambul Pediatr 2005;5(1):56–9. https://doi.org/10.1367/A04-093R.1.

36. Juckett G, Unger K. Appropriate Use of Medical Interpreters. AFP 2014;90(7):476–80.

37. Karliner LS, Jacobs EA, Chen AH, et al. Do Professional Interpreters Improve Clinical Care for Patients with Limited English Proficiency? A Systematic Review of the Literature. Health Serv Res 2007;42(2): 727–54. https://doi.org/10.1111/j.1475-6773.2006. 00629.x.

38. Jacobs B, Ryan AM, Henrichs KS, et al. Medical Interpreters in Outpatient Practice. Ann Fam Med 2018;16(1):70–6. https://doi.org/10.1370/afm.2154.

39. U.S. Department of Health and Human Services. Civil Rights. Limited English Proficiency. Available at: https://www.hhs.gov/civil-rights/for-individuals/ special-topics/limited-english-proficiency/index. html. Accessed April 21, 2022.

Racial and Ethnic Health Disparities in Dermatology

Stafford G. Brown III, MS[a,b,1], Caryn B.C. Cobb, BA[c,d,1], Valerie M. Harvey, MD, MPH[e,*]

KEYWORDS

- Racial/ethnic disparity • Health inequities • Psoriasis • Melanoma • Acne
- Hidradenitis suppurativa • Atopic dermatitis • Economic burden

KEY POINTS

- The economic burden of skin disease continues to increase, and there is a business case for eliminating health care disparities in dermatology.
- Racial and ethnic patients with psoriasis, melanoma, acne, and atopic dermatitis experience significant disparities that must be understood and addressed.
- Hidradenitis suppurativa is a disease that needs more attention to understand the prevalent disparities and their impact.

INTRODUCTION

Health disparities are differences in health or disease incidence, prevalence, severity, or disease burden that are experienced by disadvantaged populations.[1] There is significant evidence linking socially determined factors, such as housing, education level, access to food and clean water, neighborhood safety, and economic stability, on access to care and health outcomes. Health disparities are complex and multifactorial and are often linked to social and economic disadvantage. They originate from dynamic interactions of genetic, biological, environmental, social, economic, and health system–related factors.

Eliminating racial health disparities has the potential to save the United States more than $1 trillion in a 4-year period.[2] With the economic burden of health disparities in the United States projected to nearly triple from $126 billion in 2020 to $353 billion in 2050, there is a compelling business case for achieving health equity.[3] Although the economic burden of skin disease grew from $35.9 billion in 1997 to $86 billion in 2013[4–7] (Fig. 1), additional studies are needed to better understand how much of these costs was attributed to disparities in dermatologic care. There is a growing body of literature documenting disparate outcomes across cutaneous diseases, including, acne, atopic dermatitis (AD), psoriasis, hidradenitis suppurativa (HS), and melanoma.

PSORIASIS

Psoriasis is a chronic immune-mediated, inflammatory skin disease that can have a profound impact on patients' quality of life.[8] An estimated 7.55 million US adults live with psoriasis.[9] The prevalence of psoriasis is higher in white men and women at 3.6% compared with the Asian population, which is estimated to be 2.5%, the Hispanic population, at 1.9%, and the black population, at 1.5%.[9] Studies have identified ethnoracial differences in the clinical presentation of psoriasis. Asian patients have higher odds of psoriasis and erythrodermic psoriasis and lower

Dr V. Harvey is director and researcher of the Hampton University Skin of Color Research Institute, Hampton, VA, USA and a dermatologist at the Hampton Roads Center for Dermatology, Newport News, VA, USA and Virginia Beach, VA, USA.

[a] Eastern Virginia Medical School; [b] William & Mary Raymond A. Mason School of Business; [c] Hampton University Skin of Color Research Institute; [d] The Warren Alpert Medical School of Brown University; [e] Hampton Roads Center for Dermatology, 860 Omni Boulevard, Suite 114, Newport News, VA 23606, USA

[1] Contributed equally as first-authors.

* Corresponding author.

E-mail address: valerieharvey10@gmail.com

Dermatol Clin 41 (2023) 325–333
https://doi.org/10.1016/j.det.2022.10.003

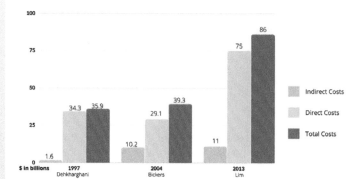

Fig. 1. The economic burden of skin disease estimates from 1997 to 2013.

frequency of inverse psoriasis compared with their white counterparts. Plaque psoriasis has been found to be the most common subtype across all ethnoracial groups.[10]

Health Care System Factors

Accessibility to effective medications may partially explain disparate psoriasis outcomes. Black patients are less likely than white patients to receive biologic treatments for their psoriasis.[11,12] In one study, 8.3% of African Americans received a disease-modifying antirheumatic drug (DMARD) and 28% received a biologic therapy, compared with 13.3% of whites, who received a DMARD, and 46.2% who received a biologic therapy. It is also difficult for Medicaid patients to have dermatologic visits covered under reimbursement models. A 2016 study found that Hispanics, blacks, and Asians had significantly higher odds (odds ratio [OR], 1.28, $P = .02$; 1.65, $P<.0001$; 2.08, $P<.0001$, respectively) of hospital admissions for psoriasis.[13] Similarly, recipients of Medicare (OR, 1.42; $P<.0001$), recipients of Medicaid (OR, 1.61; $P<.0001$), and the uninsured (OR, 3.81; $P<.0001$) experience higher rates of hospitalization for psoriasis compared with the privately insured.[13]

Economic Factors

Low socioeconomic status (SES) patients with psoriasis fare worse, consistently having a lower quality of life and work productivity than their high SES counterparts without the disease.[14–17] Non-white patients with psoriasis report the high costs of care as a significant barrier to seeking medical care.[13] Patients with higher incomes may be more able to cover expenses and also take advantage of insurance benefits to help offset the costs of treatment.[18] Furthermore, disease severity impacts job security,[18] contributing to unemployment and early retirement.[19,20]

Educational Factors

Health literacy is understanding, seeking, and using health information.[21] Suboptimal health literacy is associated with poorer health outcomes.[21] Recent multivariate analysis links low educational level to increased psoriatic disease severity.[22] Mahe and colleagues[22] found that patients with severe psoriasis of lower socioeconomic class and lower educational levels had seen fewer physicians and less frequently received a systemic treatment that those with severe psoriasis from higher SES and educational levels.

Cultural/Societal Factors

Non-white populations more frequently reported lack of culturally competent care as a barrier to seeking psoriasis treatment.[23] Hispanic and African American patients with psoriasis experience more provider-related bias, stereotyping, misdiagnosis, and delayed diagnoses compared with whites.[24] These factors may contribute to the lack of trust, lack of confidence, and fear that minority patients with psoriasis feel toward their health care providers.[24] Increasing diversity and cultural competence among health care providers enhances patient adherence, satisfaction, and outcomes of treatments.[24] Ensuring providers are clinically proficient in recognizing psoriasis across different skin types and in understanding the different cultural backgrounds of patients may improve diagnostic accuracy and strengthen the patient provider rapport.[23]

ACNE

Acne is a common skin condition with significant cutaneous and psychological sequelae. Americans are estimated to use more than 5 million physician visits for acne each year, with a direct annual cost of more than $2 billion.[5] Scarring and hyperpigmentation secondary to acne are common in skin-of-color patients and are often the chief concern.[25] Perkins and colleagues[26] found that African Americans had the highest rate of active acne, and the highest rate of combined hypertrophic and atrophic scarring compared with other groups.

Health System and Educational Factors

Barbieri and colleagues[27] found that although non-Hispanic blacks are more likely to be seen by a dermatologist, they received fewer acne prescriptions than non-Hispanic white patients. Non-Hispanic blacks and Medicaid beneficiaries were less likely to be prescribed oral antibiotics, spironolactone, and isotretinoin.[27] Medicaid patients were less likely than commercially insured patients to see a dermatologist for acne. Native Americans also have limited access to specialty care. Zullo and colleagues[28] found that 1 out of 158 participants seeking care at an Indian Health Services or tribal health care clinic was seen for acne.

Recent studies have identified flaws in the iPLEDGE system that may disproportionately burden marginalized populations (**Fig. 2**). iPLEDGE materials are above the national readability level, which may impair compliance among non-English-speaking and low-literacy patients.[29] Patients may also have limited access to computers or Internet service, which is needed to fulfill iPLEDGE requirements.[30]

Shah and colleagues[30] noted that women are twice as likely than men to prematurely terminate isotretinoin therapy. Furthermore, women who missed prescription windows resided in communities with a higher distress level than women who did not miss prescription windows. Black women are 9 times more likely than white patients to miss their prescription window.[30] The most common reasons for missed windows included insurance delays, pharmacy processing, and patient factors.[30] The mandated monthly visits are time-consuming and financially burdensome, particularly for those who cannot afford to miss time from work.[30]

In addition, Shah and colleagues[31] discovered significant lack of access to iPLEDGE pharmacies in lower-income neighborhoods and an unequal geographical distribution of pharmacies with low density in areas comprising minority inhabitants. iPLEDGE-enrolled pharmacies are more prominent in affluent neighborhoods, which may be tied to a policy termed redlining. Redlining, which dates back to the early 1900s, is based on government maps that were designed to exclude blacks and other races from purchasing homes in certain neighborhoods. Although outside the scope of this review, this policy may account for the maldistribution of pharmacies.

Economic Factors

Haider and colleagues[32] found that likelihood for referral to a dermatologist varied significantly by SES status. Similarly, this same study found that patients with acne living in urban areas had a greater likelihood of referral to a dermatologist (OR, 1.43; $P<.001$) compared with patients in a more rural area.[32] This demonstrates a clear difference in access and greater utilization of specialty care by wealthier patients with acne.

MELANOMA

From 2015 to 2018, the average incidence of melanoma (per 100,000) in the United States was 29.4% for non-Hispanic whites, 9.3% for American Indian and Alaska Natives, 4.7% for Hispanics, 1.3% for Asian and Pacific Islanders, and 1% for non-Hispanic blacks.[33] White patients had the highest percentage of stage I diagnosis at 75.9% and lowest proportion for all later stages with 12.9% diagnosed at stage II, 6.6% diagnosed at stage III, and 4.4% diagnosed at stage IV.[34] Conversely, black patients had the lowest presentation of stage I diagnosis at 52.6%, and the highest presentation for stage II at 22.82%, stage III at 13.42%, and 11.07% at stage IV.[34] From 2005 to 2009, the 5-year survival was 93% in white individuals compared with 73% in black individuals.[35] Overall, ethnic minorities are 1.96 to 3.01 times more likely to die of melanoma compared with white counterparts.[36]

Health System Factors

Recent studies have shown delays in definitive surgical intervention for melanoma in publicly insured and uninsured groups of patients.[37,38] Several studies have shown that Medicaid and uninsured patients experience delays of greater than 6 weeks from diagnosis to definitive surgery.[37,39–41] Minorities, those over 80 years old, and patients that receive care at nonacademic institutions have lower odds of undergoing excisional biopsy.[42] African Americans (OR, 0.626; $P<.001$) and lower-income patients (OR, 1; $P<.001$) (income < $63,000) are less likely to be prescribed immunotherapies compared with white patients or patients with higher incomes.[43]

Educational and Economic Factors

SES measures, such as occupation, income, educational level, insurance status, or residential status in certain neighborhoods, are determinants

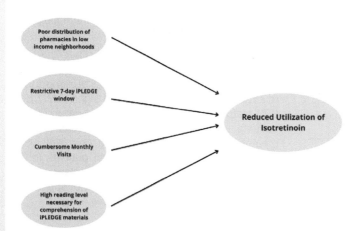

Fig. 2. Factors associated with reduced utilization of isotretinoin among minorities and those living in low-income neighborhoods.

for skin cancer screening, cutaneous melanoma incidence, and stage at diagnosis.[44,45] Many studies have demonstrated a direct correlation with incidence of cutaneous melanoma and measures of high SES.[44,46,47] Lower SES is associated with the development of thicker primary tumors (>2 mm), more advanced stage of melanoma at time of diagnosis, and increased mortalities.[44,48–52] The root cause for these disparities is multifactorial and includes lack of educational awareness about melanoma risk and melanoma presentation, and lack of access to care (**Fig. 3**). Buster and colleagues[53] noted that black patients were less likely to consider regular skin examinations important in the detection of skin cancer (OR, 0.30; P = .0009) compared with whites. Blacks and Hispanics perceive themselves as being at low risk for developing skin cancer (OR, 6.34; P<.0001; OR, 1.41; P = .1727, respectively).[53] Compared with college graduates, those with less education (measured as highest education level being high school) also perceived themselves as being at lower risk for developing skin cancer (OR, 2.076; P = .0063), worried less about developing skin cancer (OR, 1.83; P≤.0144), and had less knowledge of skin cancer prevention methods (OR, 5.00; P≤.0030).[53] Health education and promotions targeting health literacy about melanoma for minorities may provide an opportunity to change health-related attitudes, behaviors, and thus outcomes.[54]

HIDRADENITIS SUPPURATIVA

HS is a chronic inflammatory disease affecting apocrine gland–bearing skin. HS is clinically characterized by sinus tracts, abscesses, inflammatory nodules, and scarring.[55,56] Although the prevalence of HS is estimated to be 0.10% in the US population, its physical and psychosocial toll leads

to work absenteeism and reduced productivity.[57–60] A 2017 study demonstrated that population-adjusted HS prevalence is threefold higher in African Americans compared with whites.[60,61] Others report greater prevalence in young adults, women, and African Americans compared with non-Hispanic whites, with much lower rates in Hispanics.[62–65] African Americans were more likely to visit clinics for their HS.[66] A recent retrospective analysis reported increased severity in Hispanic patients when compared with non-Hispanic whites with HS. A 2022 study showed that HS has both a higher incidence/prevalence and a greater disease severity in African American people in the United States.[67]

Health Care System Factors

Disparities in HS outcomes are linked to race/ethnicity, SES, comorbid diseases, provider and patient education, and underrepresentation in clinical trials.[62,65,68] A 2021 study of black patients (5.7 mean visits) (P<.001) and Hispanic patients (4.5 mean visits) (P<.059) used outpatient services for HS more than the white patients (3.6 mean visits).[66] Black patients also present later in the disease process to tertiary care centers and have higher rates of Medicare usage (30.6%) compared with white (23%) or Hispanic (17.3%) patients with HS.[66] Less access to care to a dermatologist who is knowledgeable about HS is another systemic factor leading to inequities in marginalized populations.[69]

Economic and Educational Factors

HS is more common in both people of color and individuals from lower socioeconomic strata.[59,70] In addition to experiencing higher prevalence rates, African Americans with HS have been found to have significant health care disparities related to

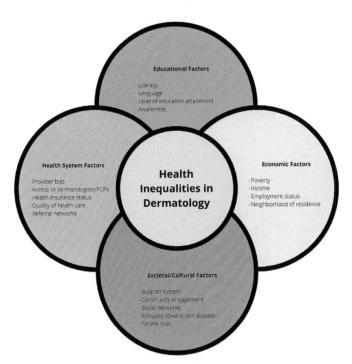

lower SES than non- African Americans patients with HS.[71] More research is needed to understand the directionality of this relationship between HS and SES.[71]

Metabolic syndrome, obesity, and smoking are risk factors for HS, which is more prevalent in women.[59,72,73] Non-Hispanic white, non-Hispanic black, and Hispanic women all have higher odds of obesity when they have a lower education level.[74] Rates of smoking are also higher in those who have only primary education.[75] Those with lower education levels also have higher odds of developing metabolic syndrome.[59,72,73] In addition to lower education attainment–related risk factors for HS, one study found that its black and Hispanic patients received less education than the white HS patients in the cohort.[66]

ATOPIC DERMATITIS

Atopic dermatitis (AD) is a common chronic pruritic inflammatory condition that follows a relapsing course. Not only does the clinical appearance and distribution of AD vary across race and ethnicity but also studies show variability in frequency and types of mutations for genes involved in barrier function and TH2 signaling pathways. AD prevalence, severity, and hospitalizations in children are higher in non-Hispanic blacks than it is in whites.[76] Among children, non-Hispanic blacks are more likely than non-Hispanic whites to visit a dermatologist for AD.[77] Blacks and Asian/Pacific

Islanders with AD are 3 to 7 times more likely than whites to seek care. Non-Hispanic blacks and Native American or Alaskan Natives experience higher levels of psychological distress and psychosocial trauma, which are both risk factors for increased severity of AD.[78,79]

Health Care System Factors

Black and Hispanic patients with AD have reported lower income, lack of transportation for work/appointments, increased need for help completing documents, and increased difficulty learning about their medical conditions when compared with white patients.[80] A recent study that surveyed patients with AD and asthma found that black patients have higher usage of Medicaid (37%) than white patients (15%).[80] In this study, 6% of participants reported having no insurance.[80] Children who have health insurance have a higher prevalence of AD compared with uninsured children ($P = .0004$), suggesting the possibility of underdiagnosis that results from decreased access to care in the latter group.[81] These barriers in access to care for lower SES patients may contribute to increased disease severity.[82]

Economic and Educational Factors

SES, exposure to air pollution and indoor allergens, and decreased access to medical care and a dermatologist are some reasons that explain the increased prevalence of AD in racial/ethnic minorities in the

United States.[80,83,84] Higher SES, heavily influenced by income, is related to increased prevalence of AD, which may be explained by detection bias or that patients with higher SES have greater access to medical care through use of insurance.[82,85,86] AD prevalence is higher in urban or metropolitan areas in the United States.[81,87] Black race (OR, 1.70; $P = .005$), household education above high school (OR, 1.61; $P = .004$), and living in an urban area (OR, 1.67; $P=.008$) were all associated with higher odds of having an AD diagnosis.[81] Lower SES is related to many risk factors (comorbidities, smoking, pollution exposure, psychological stress) for AD as well as increased AD severity.[75,82,88,89] In addition to lower household income ($P<.0001$), both maternal and paternal education levels ($P = .001$ and $P<.00001$) were associated with increased AD severity.[90]

SUMMARY

Decades of systemic and structural racism in the United States, as manifested by inequities in housing, education level, access to food and clean water, neighborhood safety, and economic instability, caused socioeconomic disparities that both create and amplify health disparities for racial groups in access to care, clinical outcomes, and erosion of trust in these communities.[88,91] As policies and strategies aimed at eliminating health care disparities are advocated for, one must be mindful of the individual level and system-level contributors. Additional studies are needed to unravel the cultural, economic, and biologic complexities that contribute to the observed inequities in outcomes among patients with skin disease.

CLINICS CARE POINTS

- Racial and ethnic disparities in dermatology outcomes are multifactorial.

- It is important to understand which educational, societal/cultural, economic, or health system factors are most impacting your patients.

- Recognizing and addressing individual-level biases toward patients is a critical step toward building trust.

- More studies are needed to better understand the social and economic drivers of poorer outcomes for minoritized populations who suffer from skin disease.

- This knowledge will inform the development of effective future interventions.

DISCLOSURE

None of the authors have any commercial or financial conflicts of interest to disclose.

REFERENCES

1. Minority health and health disparities: definitions and parameters [updated March 31, 2021]. Available at: https://www.nimhd.nih.gov/about/strategic-plan/nih-strategic-plan-definitions-and-parameters.html. Accessed June 14, 2022.
2. LaVeist TA, Gaskin D, Richard P. Estimating the economic burden of racial health inequalities in the United States. Int J Health Serv 2011;41(2):231–8.
3. Wyatt RLM, Botwinick L, Mate K, et al. Achieving health equity: a guide for health care organizations. Cambridge, Massachusetts: IHI White Paper; 2016.
4. Lim HW, Collins SAB, Resneck JS Jr, et al. The burden of skin disease in the United States. J Am Acad Dermatol 2017;76(5):958–972 e2.
5. Bickers DR, Lim HW, Margolis D, et al. The burden of skin diseases: 2004 a joint project of the American Academy of Dermatology Association and the Society for Investigative Dermatology. J Am Acad Dermatol 2006;55(3):490–500.
6. Dehkharghani S, Bible J, Chen JG, et al. The economic burden of skin disease in the United States. J Am Acad Dermatol 2003;48(4):592–9.
7. Lim HW, Collins SAB, Resneck JS Jr, et al. Contribution of health care factors to the burden of skin disease in the United States. J Am Acad Dermatol 2017;76(6):1151–1160 e21.
8. Thomsen SF, Skov L, Dodge R, et al. Socioeconomic costs and health inequalities from psoriasis: a cohort study. Dermatology 2019;235(5):372–9.
9. Armstrong AW, Mehta MD, Schupp CW, et al. Psoriasis prevalence in adults in the United States. JAMA Dermatol 2021;157(8):940–6.
10. Yan D, Afifi L, Jeon C, et al. A cross-sectional study of the distribution of psoriasis subtypes in different ethno-racial groups. Dermatol Online J 2018; 24(7).
11. Takeshita J, Eriksen WT, Raziano VT, et al. Racial differences in perceptions of psoriasis therapies: implications for racial disparities in psoriasis treatment. J Invest Dermatol 2019;139(8):1672–1679 e1.
12. Kerr GS, Qaiyumi S, Richards J, et al. Psoriasis and psoriatic arthritis in African-American patients–the need to measure disease burden. Clin Rheumatol 2015;34(10):1753–9.
13. Hsu DY, Gordon K, Silverberg JI. The inpatient burden of psoriasis in the United States. J Am Acad Dermatol 2016;75(1):33–41.
14. Seidler EM, Kimball AB. Socioeconomic disability in psoriasis. Br J Dermatol 2009;161(6):1410–2.

15. Kim GE, Seidler E, Kimball AB. A measure of chronic quality of life predicts socioeconomic and medical outcomes in psoriasis patients. J Eur Acad Dermatol Venereol 2015;29(2):249–54.

16. Jackson C, Maibach H. Ethnic and socioeconomic disparities in dermatology. J Dermatolog Treat 2016;27(3):290–1.

17. Jacobs P, Bissonnette R, Guenther LC. Socioeconomic burden of immune-mediated inflammatory diseases–focusing on work productivity and disability. J Rheumatol Suppl 2011;88:55–61.

18. Jung S, Lee SM, Suh D, et al. The association of socioeconomic and clinical characteristics with health-related quality of life in patients with psoriasis: a cross-sectional study. Health Qual Life Outcomes 2018;16(1):180.

19. Chan B, Hales B, Shear N, et al. Work-related lost productivity and its economic impact on Canadian patients with moderate to severe psoriasis. J Cutan Med Surg 2009;13(4):192–7.

20. Parisi R, Symmons DP, Griffiths CE, et al. Identification, management of P, et al. Global epidemiology of psoriasis: a systematic review of incidence and prevalence. J Invest Dermatol 2013;133(2):377–85.

21. Larsen MH, Strumse YAS, Borge CR, et al. Health literacy: a new piece of the puzzle in psoriasis care? A cross-sectional study. Br J Dermatol 2019;180(6):1506–16.

22. Mahe E, Beauchet A, Reguiai Z, et al. Socioeconomic inequalities and severity of plaque psoriasis at a first consultation in dermatology centers. Acta Derm Venereol 2017;97(5):632–8.

23. McKesey J, Berger TG, Lim HW, et al. Cultural competence for the 21st century dermatologist practicing in the United States. J Am Acad Dermatol 2017;77(6):1159–69.

24. Bray JK, Cline A, McMichael AJ, et al. Differences in healthcare barriers based on racial and/or ethnic background for patients with psoriasis. J Dermatolog Treat 2021;32(6):590–4.

25. Knutsen-Larson S, Dawson AL, Dunnick CA, et al. Acne vulgaris: pathogenesis, treatment, and needs assessment. Dermatol Clin 2012;30(1):99–106. viii-ix.

26. Perkins AC, Cheng CE, Hillebrand GG, et al. Comparison of the epidemiology of acne vulgaris among Caucasian, Asian, Continental Indian and African American women. J Eur Acad Dermatol Venereol 2011;25(9):1054–60.

27. Barbieri JS, Shin DB, Wang S, et al. Association of race/ethnicity and sex with differences in health care use and treatment for acne. JAMA Dermatol 2020;156(3):312–9.

28. Zullo SW, Maarouf M, Shi VY. Acne disparities in Native Americans. J Am Acad Dermatol 2021;85(2):499–501.

29. Howard R, Smith G. Readability of iPledge program patient education materials. J Am Acad Dermatol 2018;79(4):e69–70.

30. Shah N, Smith E, Kirkorian AY. Evaluating the barriers to isotretinoin treatment for acne vulgaris in pediatric patients. J Am Acad Dermatol 2021;85(6):1597–9.

31. Shah N, Truong M, Kirkorian AY. Relationship between sociodemographic factors and geographic distribution of pharmacies dispensing isotretinoin in Washington, DC. J Am Acad Dermatol 2020;83(3):930–3.

32. Haider A, Mamdani M, Shaw JC, et al. Socioeconomic status influences care of patients with acne in Ontario, Canada. J Am Acad Dermatol 2006;54(2):331–5.

33. Society AC. Key Statistics for Melanoma Skin Cancer. Am Cancer Soc 2022;5–7. updated January 12, 2022. Available at: https://www.cancer.org/cancer/melanoma-skin-cancer. Accessed April 25, 2022.

34. Dawes SM, Tsai S, Gittleman H, et al. Racial disparities in melanoma survival. J Am Acad Dermatol 2016;75(5):983–91.

35. Marchetti MA, Adamson AS, Halpern AC. Melanoma and racial health disparities in black individuals-facts, fallacies, and fixes. JAMA Dermatol 2021;157(9):1031–2.

36. Kundu RV, Kamaria M, Ortiz S, et al. Effectiveness of a knowledge-based intervention for melanoma among those with ethnic skin. J Am Acad Dermatol 2010;62(5):777–84.

37. Cortez JL, Vasquez J, Wei ML. The impact of demographics, socioeconomics, and health care access on melanoma outcomes. J Am Acad Dermatol 2021;84(6):1677–83.

38. Qian Y, Johannet P, Sawyers A, et al. The ongoing racial disparities in melanoma: an analysis of the Surveillance, Epidemiology, and End Results database (1975-2016). J Am Acad Dermatol 2021;84(6):1585–93.

39. Baranowski MLH, Yeung H, Chen SC, et al. Factors associated with time to surgery in melanoma: an analysis of the National Cancer Database. J Am Acad Dermatol 2019;81(4):908–16.

40. Conic RZ, Cabrera CI, Khorana AA, et al. Determination of the impact of melanoma surgical timing on survival using the National Cancer Database. J Am Acad Dermatol 2018;78(1):40–46 e7.

41. Tripathi R, Archibald LK, Mazmudar RS, et al. Racial differences in time to treatment for melanoma. J Am Acad Dermatol 2020;83(3):854–9.

42. Restrepo DJ, Huayllani MT, Boczar D, et al. Biopsy type disparities in patients with melanoma: who receives the standard of care? Anticancer Res 2019;39(11):6359–63.

43. Alicea GM, Rebecca VW. Un-Fair Skin: racial disparities in acral melanoma research. Nat Rev Cancer 2022;22(3):127–8.

44. Harvey VM, Patel H, Sandhu S, et al. Social determinants of racial and ethnic disparities in cutaneous melanoma outcomes. Cancer Control 2014;21(4):343–9.

45. Pollitt RA, Clarke CA, Swetter SM, et al. The expanding melanoma burden in California hispanics: Importance of socioeconomic distribution, histologic subtype, and anatomic location. Cancer 2011; 117(1):152–61.

46. Rouhani P, Hu S, Kirsner RS. Melanoma in Hispanic and black Americans. Cancer Control 2008;15(3): 248–53.

47. Wich LG, Ma MW, Price LS, et al. Impact of socioeconomic status and sociodemographic factors on melanoma presentation among ethnic minorities. J Community Health 2011;36(3):461–8.

48. Cormier JN, Xing Y, Ding M, et al. Ethnic differences among patients with cutaneous melanoma. Arch Intern Med 2006;166(17):1907–14.

49. Stubblefield J, Kelly B. Melanoma in non-Caucasian populations. Surg Clin North Am 2014;94(5): 1115–26, ix.

50. Hu S, Parmet Y, Allen G, et al. Disparity in melanoma: a trend analysis of melanoma incidence and stage at diagnosis among whites, Hispanics, and blacks in Florida. Arch Dermatol 2009;145(12): 1369–74.

51. Ortiz CA, Goodwin JS, Freeman JL. The effect of socioeconomic factors on incidence, stage at diagnosis and survival of cutaneous melanoma. Med Sci Monit 2005;11(5):RA163–72.

52. Pollitt RA, Swetter SM, Johnson TM, et al. Examining the pathways linking lower socioeconomic status and advanced melanoma. Cancer 2012;118(16): 4004–13.

53. Buster KJ, You Z, Fouad M, et al. Skin cancer risk perceptions: a comparison across ethnicity, age, education, gender, and income. J Am Acad Dermatol 2012;66(5):771–9.

54. Wu T, Wang X, Zhao S, et al. Socioeconomic determinants of melanoma-related health literacy and attitudes among college students in China: a population-based cross-sectional study. Front Public Health 2021;9:743368.

55. Jemec GB. Clinical practice. Hidradenitis suppurativa. N Engl J Med 2012;366(2):158–64.

56. Tricarico PM, Boniotto M, Genovese G, et al. An integrated approach to unravel hidradenitis suppurativa etiopathogenesis. Front Immunol 2019;10:892.

57. Deckers IE, Kimball AB. The handicap of hidradenitis suppurativa. Dermatol Clin 2016;34(1):17–22.

58. Pinard J, Vleugels RA, Joyce C, et al. Hidradenitis suppurativa burden of disease tool: pilot testing of a disease-specific quality of life questionnaire. J Am Acad Dermatol 2018;78(1):215–217 e2.

59. Lee DE, Clark AK, Shi VY. Hidradenitis suppurativa: disease burden and etiology in skin of color. Dermatology 2017;233(6):456–61.

60. Garg A, Kirby JS, Lavian J, et al. Sex- and age-adjusted population analysis of prevalence estimates for hidradenitis suppurativa in the United States. JAMA Dermatol 2017;153(8):760–4.

61. Okeke CAV, Perry JD, Simmonds FC, et al. Clinical trials and skin of color: the example of hidradenitis suppurativa. Dermatology 2022;238(1):180–4.

62. Vaidya T, Vangipuram R, Alikhan A. Examining the race-specific prevalence of hidradenitis suppurativa at a large academic center; results from a retrospective chart review. Dermatol Online J 2017; 23(6):1–2.

63. Garg A, Wertenteil S, Baltz R, et al. Prevalence estimates for hidradenitis suppurativa among children and adolescents in the United States: a gender- and age-adjusted population analysis. J Invest Dermatol 2018;138(10):2152–6.

64. Sachdeva M, Shah M, Alavi A. Race-specific prevalence of hidradenitis suppurativa. J Cutan Med Surg 2021;25(2):177–87.

65. Vlassova N, Kuhn D, Okoye GA. Hidradenitis suppurativa disproportionately affects African Americans: a single-center retrospective analysis. Acta Derm Venereol 2015;95(8):990–1.

66. Kilgour JM, Li S, Sarin KY. Hidradenitis suppurativa in patients of color is associated with increased disease severity and healthcare utilization: a retrospective analysis of 2 U.S. cohorts. JAAD Int 2021;3: 42–52.

67. Cullen MR, Lemeshow AR, Russo LJ, et al. Disease-specific health disparities: a targeted review focusing on race and ethnicity. Healthcare (Basel). 2022;10(4).

68. Price KN, Hsiao JL, Shi VY. Race and ethnicity gaps in global hidradenitis suppurativa clinical trials. Dermatology 2021;237(1):97–102.

69. Shukla N, Paul M, Halley M, et al. Identifying barriers to care and research in hidradenitis suppurativa: findings from a patient engagement event. Br J Dermatol 2020;182(6):1490–2.

70. Deckers IE, Janse IC, van der Zee HH, et al. Hidradenitis suppurativa (HS) is associated with low socioeconomic status (SES): a cross-sectional reference study. J Am Acad Dermatol 2016;75(4): 755–759 e1.

71. Soliman YS, Hoffman LK, Guzman AK, et al. African American patients with hidradenitis suppurativa have significant health care disparities: a retrospective study. J Cutan Med Surg 2019;23(3):334–6.

72. Miller IM, McAndrew RJ, Hamzavi I. Prevalence, risk factors, and comorbidities of hidradenitis suppurativa. Dermatol Clin 2016;34(1):7–16.

73. Miller IM. Co-morbidities in inflammatory dermatological diseases. Psoriasis, hidradenitis suppurativa,

and cardiovascular risk factors. Dan Med J 2015; 62(9).

74. Ogden CL, Fakhouri TH, Carroll MD, et al. Prevalence of obesity among adults, by household income and education - United States, 2011-2014. MMWR Morb Mortal Wkly Rep 2017;66(50):1369–73.

75. Mahdaviazad H, Foroutan R, Masoompour SM. Prevalence of tobacco smoking and its socioeconomic determinants: tobacco smoking and its determinants. Clin Respir J 2022;16(3):208–15.

76. Castells M. Race and allergy: are we that different? Ann Allergy Asthma Immunol 2019;122(5):439–40.

77. Fischer AH, Shin DB, Margolis DJ, et al. Racial and ethnic differences in health care utilization for childhood eczema: an analysis of the 2001-2013 Medical Expenditure Panel Surveys. J Am Acad Dermatol 2017;77(6):1060–7.

78. Oh SH, Bae BG, Park CO, et al. Association of stress with symptoms of atopic dermatitis. Acta Derm Venereol 2010;90(6):582–8.

79. Lugovic-Mihic L, Mestrovic-Stefekov J, Pondeljak N, et al. Psychological stress and atopic dermatitis severity following the COVID-19 pandemic and an earthquake. Psychiatr Danub 2021;33(3):393–401.

80. Bukstein DA, Friedman A, Gonzalez Reyes E, et al. Impact of social determinants on the burden of asthma and eczema: results from a US patient survey. Adv Ther 2022;39(3):1341–58.

81. Shaw TE, Currie GP, Koudelka CW, et al. Eczema prevalence in the United States: data from the 2003 National Survey of Children's Health. J Invest Dermatol 2011;131(1):67–73.

82. Chung J, Simpson EL. The socioeconomics of atopic dermatitis. Ann Allergy Asthma Immunol 2019;122(4):360–6.

83. Croce EA, Levy ML, Adamson AS, et al. Reframing racial and ethnic disparities in atopic dermatitis in Black and Latinx populations. J Allergy Clin Immunol 2021;148(5):1104–11.

84. Chiesa Fuxench ZC, Block JK, Boguniewicz M, et al. Atopic dermatitis in America study: a cross-sectional study examining the prevalence and disease burden of atopic dermatitis in the US adult population. J Invest Dermatol 2019;139(3):583–90.

85. Silverberg JI, Hanifin JM. Adult eczema prevalence and associations with asthma and other health and demographic factors: a US population-based study. J Allergy Clin Immunol 2013;132(5):1132–8.

86. Torfi Y, Bitarafan N, Rajabi M. Impact of socioeconomic and environmental factors on atopic eczema and allergic rhinitis: a cross sectional study. EXCLI J 2015;14:1040–8.

87. McKenzie C, Silverberg JI. The prevalence and persistence of atopic dermatitis in urban United States children. Ann Allergy Asthma Immunol 2019;123(2):173–178 e1.

88. Martinez A, de la Rosa R, Mujahid M, et al. Structural racism and its pathways to asthma and atopic dermatitis. J Allergy Clin Immunol 2021;148(5): 1112–20.

89. Adler NE, Newman K. Socioeconomic disparities in health: pathways and policies. Health Aff (Millwood) 2002;21(2):60–76.

90. Silverberg JI, Simpson EL. Associations of childhood eczema severity: a US population-based study. Dermatitis 2014;25(3):107–14.

91. Tackett KJ, Jenkins F, Morrell DS, et al. Structural racism and its influence on the severity of atopic dermatitis in African American children. Pediatr Dermatol 2020;37(1):142–6.

History of Race in America

Ellen N. Pritchett, MD, MPH[a], Rebecca Vasquez, MD[b],*

KEYWORDS

- Race • Ethnicity • History • America • Black • African • Native American • Mexican

KEY POINTS

- Race, as a social construct, emerged during the colonial period and used visible phenotypic characteristics and ancestry to justify systems of oppression and privilege.
- The legacy of these inequitable systems is still felt today and shape opportunities in housing, education, economic stability, and health care (also known as the social determinants of health).
- It is important to recognize how these inequitable systems operate and mitigate their impact on racial and ethnic health disparities.

INTRODUCTION

Before the 1500s, the term "race" was used to identify groups of people with kinship or connection. Members of the same household or those who shared a common ancestor were considered of the same race.[1,2] With the rise of global capitalism backed by slavery, Manifest Destiny, and colonialism, the meaning of race began to change. Theories that developed during the Enlightenment period, which emphasized science and reason over faith and superstition, strongly influenced the American colonies during the eighteenth century, and there was a push in the scientific community to categorize the natural world using reason. Elaborate hierarchical systems that emphasized the similarities and inherent differences between species and subgroups were developed. The idea of race was fitted into the same mold.[1]

Attempts to classify human populations into races by scientists started with Carl Linnaeus in 1735. He divided the races into the following four groups: White (Europeans), who were "acute, gentle, and inventive;" Red (Native Americans), who were "obstinate, merry, and free;" Dark (Asians), who were "stiff, haughty, and avaricious;" and Black (Africans), who were "phlegmatic, indolent, and negligent".[3] Race, consequently, became less about kinship groups and more about pseudoscientific racial distinctions, such as identifying groups of people by physical traits, appearance, and characteristics.[1,2]

European settlers in America and, consequently, the founding fathers of American democracy began using these pseudoscientific racial distinctions among the population to justify enslaving and discriminating against whole groups of people. Race, as a social construct, would become codified into law and help structure an inegalitarian society. Native Americans, Africans, and their descendants, regardless of their cultural similarities or differences, were forced into categories separate from Whites. Mexican Americans were classified as White; however, their de jure status was undermined by White-American prejudice precluding their entitlement to many of the White social privileges.[4] Chinese, Japanese, and Jewish immigrants were viewed as racial or ethnic others and were largely excluded from political rights, higher education, and occasionally, even society.[4–6]

Herein, we discuss select periods in history (**Fig. 1**) to demonstrate how racial ideologies shaped public attitudes and policies during that time and resulted in the marginalization of certain groups. The repercussions of this are still felt today through persistent inequities in housing, employment, education, and health care also known as the social determinants of health—the primary

[a] Department of Dermatology, Howard University College of Medicine, 2041 Georgia Avenue NW, Towers Building, Suite 4300, Washington, DC 20060, USA; [b] Department of Dermatology, University of Texas Southwestern Medical Center, Dallas, TX, USA
* Corresponding author. 5939 Harry Hines Boulevard, Dallas, TX 75235.
E-mail address: rebecca.vasquez@utsouthwestern.edu

Dermatol Clin 41 (2023) 335–343
https://doi.org/10.1016/j.det.2022.08.004

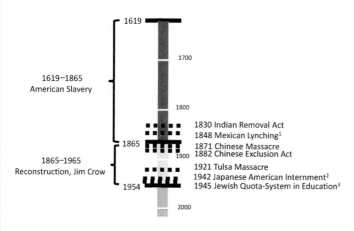

Fig. 1. Historical timeline of events. 1. Lynching rate of Mexicans was highest between 1848 and 1879 (during the aftermath of the US-Mexican War) but took place until the early part of twentieth century. 2. Japanese American Internment camps remained for the duration of the war from 1942 to 1945. 3. Quota systems to limit access of Jews in medical schools were in place by the early 1920s but firmly entrenched by 1945. (Available at: https://blogs.berkeley.edu/2018/10/25/the-american-pipe-bomb/5a9ee7e77add3-image/)

drivers of racial and ethnic health disparities in medicine.

ORIGINS OF CHATTEL SLAVERY (1619–1865)

The United States has a long history as a slave-holding republic.[5] With the arrival of approximately 20 Africans from the Ndongo Kingdom in West Central Africa (modern-day Angola) that were captured from a Portuguese slave ship, Virginia became acquainted with the transatlantic slave trade in 1619.[7] Although still under debate, historians argue that labor in early Colonial America included both those of European and African descent, and servitude in the early 1600s was not always hereditary with the possibility of freedom either through the end of a contract or manumission.[8] In addition, Africans labored and socialized alongside European indentured servants.

The first large-scale rebellion in the North American Colonies, or Bacon's Rebellion of 1676, became a turning point for the status and rights of people of African descent in Virginia and planted the seeds of chattel slavery (a form of slavery in the United States where enslaved people were legally considered as personal property).[9] The conflict arose after Nathanial Bacon, a wealthy White property owner, wanted to take Native Americans' land. Bacon organized a militia of Black and White indentured servants and enslaved Black people to attack Native Americans.[10] After months of conflict between Bacon and Governor Berkeley of Virginia, Bacon's militia captured Jamestown, Virginia and burned it to the ground.[10] The alliance between White and Black indentured servants and the threat of insurrection alarmed the colonial leaders.[10] Consequently, the solution was to divide the two groups and make legal distinctions between Black and White.[9] The long-term effects would include the Virginia Slaves Codes of 1705

that firmly established race-based slavery in the United States.[11]

In 1794, Eli Whitney successfully patented the cotton gin; this development led to the growth of slavery and the geographic expansion of the United States. The cotton gin made cotton processing less laborious, motivating planters to grow larger crops for greater profit, which required additional cheap sources of labor.[12] Although the transatlantic slave trade was outlawed in 1808, the domestic trade of enslaved people within the United States, known as the second middle passage, became more substantial during this time, and the number of enslaved people continued to rise.[13] Enslaved people were forced to migrate from the Upper South tobacco plantations to the new Lower South cotton plantations,[14] thereby causing the dissolution of thousands of enslaved families.[15]

Enslavers moved southwest in search of new farmland for cotton (some historians believe this prompted the Indian Removal Act of 1830—to be discussed later). For the North, the cotton increase provided a steady supply of raw materials for textile manufacturing.[13,16] By the mid- nineteenth century, cotton was America's leading export and slavery became central to the development and growth of the economy.[16] Also during this period, racism became institutionalized; additional laws were enacted to limit the social, political, and economic mobility of enslaved people and to uphold racial hierarchies of White superiority and Black inferiority, thereby ensuring the financial prosperity of enslavers.

CIVIL WAR (1861–1865), RECONSTRUCTION (1865-1877), AND JIM CROW (1877-1965)

In the North, growing opposition to slavery's expansion into new territories alarmed Southerners that slavery, the backbone of their economy, was in jeopardy.[17] Abraham Lincoln was elected in 1860 as the first Republican president on an antislavery platform.[15] These factors caused several states of the South to secede and form a new nation, the Confederate States of America. The fighting started in April 1861 at Fort Sumter in South Carolina and ended in 1865. Ultimately, the Confederacy and the South's infrastructure were destroyed, more than 600,000 were killed, slavery was abolished and the United States entered into the Reconstruction Era.[17]

During the Reconstruction Era of 1865 to 1877, federal laws provided civil rights protections for formerly enslaved people and the minority of Blacks who were free before the war. On December 6, 1865, slavery was abolished, except as a punishment for crime, with the ratification of the 13th Amendment of the Constitution. In 1868, the passage of the 14th Amendment granted citizenship to persons born or naturalized in the United States, including formerly enslaved people, and equal protection under the law to citizens. In 1870, the 15th Amendment granted the right to vote to Black men.

Unfortunately, with the rise of these federal gains in political freedom, new restrictive methods were created to undermine them and ensure that Black people would still be used as a cheap source of labor.[18] New laws known as Black Codes were enacted at local and state levels to prevent the social and economic mobility that might be acquired from the federal laws. These laws vary by state, but they all placed restrictions on property ownership, the right to own weapons, testifying in court, and learning to read, among other limitations.[19] A defining feature was vagrancy statutes, in which unemployed Black people would be arrested and forced to hard labor.[19] Voting was restricted through the use of poll taxes (ie, a fee to vote), grandfather clauses (ie, voting restricted to male descendants of persons who were eligible to vote before 1866 or 1867), the White primary (ie, only White voters permitted) and literacy tests.[20] The Ku Klux Klan, which was founded in 1866 in Pulaski, Tennessee to restore White supremacy by using intimidation and violence against Blacks and White supporters, was used to enforce these Black Codes.[19] These Black Codes set the precedent for Jim Crow laws.

The Compromise of 1876, which led to the removal of the troops from the South, ended the Reconstruction period and led to Jim Crow laws. These laws, named after the minstrel routine "Jump, Jim Crow," enforced racial segregation in public transportation and other public facilities and led to widespread disenfranchisement and institutionalized disadvantages for Black people.[21]

These laws were legitimized in the 1896 Supreme Court case of *Plessy v. Ferguson*.[20] Homer Plessy was 7 of 8 White and 1 of 8 Black. He sat in the Whites' only car of a Louisiana train and was arrested.[20] The court declared that "separate-but-equal" facilities were constitutional and did not violate the equal protection clause of the 14th Amendment.[20] The "separate but equal" doctrine was then applied to other public facilities and had devastating, poverty-concentrating effects. Facilities for Black people were inferior, underfunded, and oftentimes nonexistent as compared with those for White people.[22] In the 1930s, the Federal Housing Administration furthered segregation efforts by implementing redlining policies that assigned risk ratings to certain neighborhoods and refused to insure mortgages in Black, lower class, or immigrant neighborhoods.[23] Violence was instrumental for Jim Crow as a method of social control and intimidation, and the most extreme form was lynching.[20]

One of the worst acts of racial violence against Black people occurred in the Greenwood District of Tulsa, Oklahoma between May 31, 1921 and June 1, 1921.[24] Referred to as the Black Wall Street, the Greenwood District was one of the wealthiest Black communities in the United States. Dick Rowland, a Black teenager, got into an elevator in the Drexel Building that was operated by Sarah Page, a White woman. Page screamed and the police were called. Rowland fled, and the next morning he was arrested. Although it is uncertain what happened in the elevator, the following afternoon, the Tulsa Tribune published a front-page story indicating that Rowland attempted to sexually assault Page.[24] This story prompted groups of White Tulsans to commit acts of violence against Black Tulsans, including looting and burning of homes, churches, doctor's offices, grocery stores, a public library, and other Black-owned businesses.[24] It is estimated that up to 300 people, mostly Black, died, and the Greenwood District was destroyed.[25] Approximately $4 million worth of property damage claims were submitted to insurance companies. Unfortunately, they were all denied.[25]

In 1954, the Supreme Court case of *Brown v. Board of Education* reversed the *Plessy v. Ferguson* ruling by declaring segregation in public schools unconstitutional and by extension segregation of other public facilities. Generations of resistance to segregation culminated in the Civil Rights movement; and as a result, new legislation, including the Civil Rights Act of 1964, the Voting Rights Act of 1965, and the Fair Housing Act of 1968 were passed.[21] These laws aimed to eliminate discrimination in employment, voting, and housing and essentially ended the Jim Crow era.

NATIVE AMERICANS AND THE INDIAN REMOVAL ACT OF 1830

Against the backdrop of Manifest Destiny in the nineteenth century and enslavers' quest for new farmland for cotton, Native Americans were forcibly expelled from their ancestral homelands in the south to the western lands of the United States to accommodate European settlers under the banner of the Indian Removal Act of 1830.[26]

President Andrew Jackson (who called for Indian removal during the State of the Union address in 1829) sincerely believed that this population transfer was a "wise and humane policy" that would save the Native Americans from "utter annihilation".[27]

Yet, in the decades immediately before the time of removal in the 1830s and 1840s, the Native Americans of the southern tribes had developed extensive economic ties with the European American colonizers and, out of necessity, began to adapt to the American settler culture around them. Because of this adaptation, the southern tribes (including the Choctaw, Chickasaw, Seminole, Creek, and Cherokee people) became known as the "Five Civilized Tribes" (a term Native American historians no longer use).[28,29]

The land occupied by these Five Tribes (located in parts of Georgia, Alabama, North Carolina, Florida, and Tennessee) was valuable, and it grew to be more coveted as European settlers flooded the region.[30] To European settlers in America, the tribes were hindering progress and America's Manifest Destiny.[31]

By the end of Jackson's Presidency, his administration had negotiated almost 70 removal treaties.[32] Native American participation in removal was meant to be voluntary, and the law required the US government to negotiate fairly with the tribes. However, this was not often the result. Many tribes were forcibly removed from their lands, in particular the Cherokee, Choctaw, Creek, Chickasaw, and Seminole.

Of the individual treaties signed following the Indian Removal Act, the first was between the United States and the Choctaw Nation in 1830. Between 1831 and 1834, most members of this nation were forced westward in appalling conditions. Because federal expenditures for removal were inadequate, there were food shortages, unsatisfactory means of transportation, and sparse clothing or blankets. At least a quarter of the Choctaw Nation died before they reached the new Indian Territory in modern-day Oklahoma. A similar fate befell the other nations.[33,34]

The Cherokees, the most numerous of the Five Tribes, resisted deportation, arguing the case against the highest US tribunals including the Senate and the Supreme Court. However, they were unsuccessful. The Treaty of New Echota, signed on December 29, 1835, ceded all Cherokee territory to the United States and they were forced to leave by 1839. Between 1838 and 1839, members of this nation moved westward in dreadful conditions and approximately one-quarter of the Cherokees perished between 1838 and 1839.[31,34]

The series of forced migrations, now known as the Trail of Tears, and the constant cultural assimilation accompanied by the unjust treatment of Native Americans by the United States have been described as cultural and even de facto genocide.[31,35,36] Although the Trail of Tears is perhaps the best-known instance of forced relocation, the government also implemented many other forced removals, including the infamous Navajo Long Walk[37] and the Japanese American Internment.[38,39]

Native American removal not only forced native people westward, but also facilitated the expansion of slavery in the Deep South. Nearly 25 million acres of land became available to European settlers in America for cotton production. As a result, treaties and policies created to enforce Indian removal accommodated and expanded the institution of chattel slavery.[31]

MEXICAN LYNCHING OF 1800S

Manifest Destiny also fueled colonial expansion into the Southwest and Western regions of what is now the United States.[26] Vigilantism and brutal oppression (tantamount to state-sanctioned terrorism) by way of mob violence allowed European Americans to establish their colonial control of the American West and helped facilitate the widespread dispossession of land that was previously owned by Mexicans.[4,40] As a result, tens of thousands of Mexican Americans in New Mexico lost their communally owned lands and, consequently, became wage laborers that often had to migrate out of the region seasonally to earn a living.[40]

Without proper legal authorities, European Americans often took the law into their own hands. Vigilantism, at least initially, served a legitimate purpose in the settlement of the American West, preserving order and paving the way for a formal legal system. But even after the arrival of official legal courts, vigilante committees persisted in their activities. European Americans refused to recognize the legitimacy of legal courts when they were controlled or influenced by Mexicans.[4] These vigilante committees showed little respect for the legal rights of Mexicans, executing them in disproportionately large numbers. Still, only a small number of Mexican lynching victims—64 out of 597—met their fate at the hands of vigilante committees and most of them were executed by mobs that denied the accused even the semblance of a trial.

Between 1848 and 1928, mobs lynched greater than 500 Mexicans. The locations of most of these cases were Texas (282), California (188), Arizona (59), and New Mexico (49). Historians discovered a surprising lynching incidence rate of 473 per 100,000 between 1848 and 1879 during the aftermath of the US–Mexican War. By the turn of the twentieth century, the rate had reduced to 27.4 lynching victims per 100,000. As a comparison, during the same period, lynching rates for African Americans in the South varied from North Carolina's 11 per 100,000 to Alabama's 32.4 per 100,000.[4]

Mexican lynching not only occurred in areas where there was a fully operating legal system but often involved the active collusion of law officers. The most systematic abuse was by the Texas Rangers. Although the exact number of those murdered by Rangers is unknown, historians estimate it to be in the hundreds and even thousands.[4]

Although not exclusive to Black and Mexican people living in America, other racial and ethnic groups were also victims of mob violence and lynching as documented in the Chinese Massacre of 1871. However, Black and Mexican Americans lived with the threat of lynching throughout the second half of the nineteenth and the first half of the twentieth centuries.[4]

CHINESE MASSACRE OF 1871 AND THE CHINESE EXCLUSION ACT OF 1882

The Chinese first immigrated to the United States during the California Gold Rush in 1848. They were a substantial part of the labor force that built the economic infrastructure of the American West, and they were instrumental in constructing the Transcontinental Railroad. As the number of Chinese laborers increased, so did the strength of anti-Chinese sentiment, particularly among US workers.[41–43] The racist trope of "yellow peril" developed. There were fears that Chinese workers undercut wages by working for lower pay, endangered America's westward expansion and were a threat to a free White republic, although they composed only 0.002% of the US population at that time.[42,43]

This hostile climate fueled the Chinese Massacre of 1871 in which approximately 18 people or 10% of Los Angeles, California's Chinese population of 172 were killed.[44] Two members of rival Chinese groups had a gunfight over a woman, which resulted in a wounded police officer and the death of a White civilian.[44] This sparked a riot that involved a mob of people looting homes and businesses and assaulting Chinese residents. The Chinese Massacre of 1871 was one of several riots and killings, which include the 1885 Rock Springs Massacre in Wyoming.

Amid this racially motivated violence, growing anti-Chinese sentiment, and the economic depression of the West, the US government passed the Chinese Exclusion Act. This Act was the first in American history to restrict immigration based solely on nationality.[41–43] It prohibited the entry of Chinese laborers to the United States for a period of 10 years and denied US citizenship through naturalization. Several racially motivated immigration laws were subsequently put into place that reinforced the Chinese Exclusion Act. In 1888, the Scott Act made reentry to the United States after a visit to China impossible, even for long-term residents.[45] In 1892, the Geary Act extended the Chinese Exclusion Act for another 10 years, and in 1902 the Chinese Exclusion Act was made permanent.[45] It was not until 1943 (nearly 60 years after it was enacted) when the United States and China were allies against Japan during World War II that the Exclusion Act was finally repealed.[45]

JAPANESE AMERICAN INTERNMENT

Anti-Japanese actions became more pervasive in 1905.[46] They arose from prejudices against the Chinese, increased Japanese immigration, and Japan's victory over Russia.[46] Anti-Japanese organizations, such as the Asiatic Exclusion League, were formed, schools were segregated under the Jim Crow doctrine of "separate but equal", and attacks on individuals and businesses occurred.[46] In addition, laws prohibiting immigration and property ownership were enacted.[46] These factors, in addition to negative racial stereotypes, influenced the Japanese American forced relocation or internment shortly following the attack on Pearl Harbor during World War II.[46]

President Franklin D. Roosevelt established Japanese internment camps through Executive Order 9066.[38] Approximately 120,000 people of Japanese descent (defined as 1/16th Japanese or more), the majority of whom were US citizens, were forcibly removed from their homes and incarcerated in camps.[38,39] These camps were located in remote areas of California, Arizona, Wyoming, Colorado, Utah, and Arkansas.[38] Executive Order 9066 also called for the compulsory relocation of some Italian and German Americans.[47]

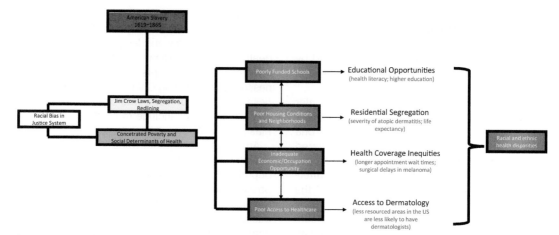

Fig. 2. Legacy of structural racism and impact on health disparities. (*Adapted from* Churchwell K, Elkind MSV, Benjamin RM, Carson AP, Chang EK, Lawrence W, Mills A, Odom TM, Rodriguez CJ, Rodriguez F, Sanchez E, Sharrief AZ, Sims M, Williams O; American Heart Association. Call to Action: Structural Racism as a Fundamental Driver of Health Disparities: A Presidential Advisory From the American Heart Association. Circulation. 2020 Dec 15;142(24):e454-e468.)

Japanese Americans were thought to be spies or pose a security risk despite a lack of evidence that they presented a danger to the United States.[38] They were only given a few days to liquidate their assets, often at a fraction of their true value, gather the possessions they could carry, and report to a temporary assembly center while awaiting transport to their assigned internment camps.[38] Many remained for the duration of the war from 1942 to 1945.

In 1976, President Gerald Ford repealed Executive Order 9066. In 1988, a formal apology was issued by Congress and the Civil Liberties Act was passed, which awarded $20,000 in reparations to more than 80,000 surviving Japanese Americans.[38]

JEWISH DISCRIMINATION AND QUOTAS IN US MEDICAL EDUCATION

In response to the massive wave of Russian Jewish immigrants at the beginning of the twentieth century, and the interest of these immigrants and their children in medical education, quotas restricting the access of Jewish students and physicians to medical school and postgraduate training were put into place, respectively.[48,49] In 1920, for example, there were 214 Jewish students enrolled in medical schools in New York state. By 1940, there were 108. In an era in which it was estimated that 32% to 50% of US medical school applicants were Jews, the medical historian Henry Sigerist concluded that these applicants were "subject to a tacit, but nevertheless highly effective, quota-system and in most schools the number of Jewish students rarely [exceeded] 10 per cent ..."[48,49] The quotas ended well after

World War II due to changes in societal attitudes and both government and private social action.[49]

SUMMARY

Throughout the history of race in America, structural racism has routinely advantaged Whites and disenfranchised other racial and ethnic groups through a variety of practices. Slavery was legalized. Jim Crow laws permitted racial segregation. The Chinese Exclusion Act prohibited the immigration of Chinese laborers. The Indian Removal Act forcibly removed Native American people from their land. The Japanese American Internment forcibly removed people from their homes and incarcerated them in camps, and Jewish immigrants were restricted access to higher education.[6] Lynching was widespread and used as a method to control, terrorize, and enforce legal systems of racial oppression, especially toward Black Americans and Mexican Americans during the second half of the nineteenth and the first half of the twentieth centuries. Although the authors have only discussed a few groups and selected historical events in this article, we acknowledge that other people of color in the United States—who have not been mentioned—have also been the target of health-harming racial discrimination, combined with antiimmigrant and religious (eg, anti-Muslim) discrimination.

The legacy of these discriminatory laws, economic systems, and social hierarchies that have defined structural racism still has a profound impact on health inequities today. For example, poorly funded schools contribute to differences in educational opportunities thereby affecting health literacy[50] and educational attainment[51]; poor housing conditions in concentrated areas perpetuate residential segregation that can affect a variety of health outcomes from the severity of atopic dermatitis in Black children[52] to overall life expectancy in Black adults[5]; inadequate employment opportunities can determine health coverage (with more restrictive plans like Medicaid associated with longer appointment wait times[53] and surgical delays in melanoma[54]); living in less-resourced areas can disproportionately affect access to dermatology for communities of color (where dermatologists are more likely to be located in well-resourced urban areas[55]) **(Fig. 2)**. This history of codified racism in the United States has led national medical organizations to declare racism a threat to public health, to the advancement of health equity and a barrier to appropriate medical care.[56] Strategies to help mitigate its effects start with acknowledging that racism within health care (and medical research) harms marginalized communities and supporting policy to combat racism and its deleterious effects.[56]

CLINICS CARE POINTS

- Although civil rights laws were passed in the 1960s, historical practices (eg, approximately 246 years of slavery and 100 years of Jim Crow) and systemic racism continue to drive present-day inequities in social determinants of health that produce racial and ethnic health disparities.

- It is our duty, as physicians, to recognize how structural racism operates in health care and advocate for the advancement of health equity.

- Systematic interventions at multiple levels, including community engagement, health care policies and practices, and allyship among racial and ethnic groups offer promise to modify health disparities.

DISCLOSURE

The authors have no disclosures to report.

REFERENCES

1. Talking About Race: Historical Foundations of Race. In. National Museum of African American History and Culture Smithsonian.
2. Hudson N. "Nation to "Race": The Origin of Racial Classification in Eighteenth-Century Thought. Eighteenth-Century Stud 1996;29(3):247–64.
3. Kelly AP, Taylor SC, Lim HW, et al. Taylor and Kelly's dermatology for Skin of color. 2nd ed. McGraw-Hill Education.; 2016.
4. Carrigan WD, Webb C. The Lynching of Persons of Mexican Origin or Descent in the United States, 1848 to 1928. J Social Hist 2003;37(2):411–38.
5. Bailey ZD, Krieger N, Agenor M, et al. Structural racism and health inequities in the USA: evidence and interventions. Lancet 2017;389(10077):1453–63.
6. Sokoloff L. The rise and decline of the Jewish quota in medical school admissions. Bull N Y Acad Med 1992;68(4):497–518.
7. Thornton J. Africa and Africans in the making of the Atlantic world, 1400–1800. Cambridge University Press; 1998.
8. Vaughan AT. The Origins Debate: Slavery and Racism in Seventeenth-Century Virginia. Va Mag Hist Biogr 1989;97(3):311–54.
9. Rice J. Bacon's rebellion in Indian Country101. Oxford University Press/USA.; 2014.
10. Inventing Black and White. Facing History and Ourselves Web site. Available at: https://www.facinghistory.org/holocaust-and-human-behavior/chapter-2/inventing-black-and-white. Accessed May 17, 2022.
11. Slavery in America. Ferris State University. Available at: https://www.ferris.edu/HTMLS/news/jimcrow/timeline/slavery.htm. Accessed May 18, 2022.
12. Riggs T. Cotton Gin Turns Cotton into Leading Cash Crop, Increases Demand for Slave Labor. In: Riggs T. ed., Gale Encyclopedia of U.S. Economic History. 2015, Vol 1. 2nd edn, Gale: Farmington Hills, MI, p.306–7.
13. Hillstrom K, Hillstrom LC. Slavery and the American South. In: Baker LW, editor. Am Civil War Reference Libr 2000;3:1–14.
14. Morabia A. Slavery, Work, and Racism in America: A Review of Four Books. Am J Public Health 2019; 109(10):1312–4.
15. Halpern R, Lago ED. Slavery and Emancipation. In: John Wiley & Sons, Incorporated. 2002. Available at: http://ebookcentral.proquest.com/lib/howard/detail.action?docID=351441.
16. Bailey R. The Other Side of Slavery: Black Labor, Cotton, and Textile Industrialization in Great Britain and the United States. Agric Hist 1994;68(2):35–50.
17. Civil War. History.com. 2009. Available at: https://www.history.com/topics/american-civil-war/american-civil-war-history. Accessed May 17, 2022.
18. Black Codes. History.com. 2010. Available at: https://www.history.com/topics/black-history/black-codes. Accessed May 17 2022.
19. Black Code. Ferris State University. Available at: https://www.ferris.edu/HTMLS/news/jimcrow/links/misclink/blackcode.htm. Accessed May 17, 2022.
20. Pilgrim D. Using Racist Memorabilia to Teach Tolerance and Promote Social Justice. In: PM Press.

2015. Available at: http://ebookcentral.proquest.com/lib/howard/detail.action?docID=4306903.

21. Jim Crow and segregation: classroom materials at the library of congress. The Library of Congress. Available at: https://www.loc.gov/classroom-materials/jim-crow-segregation/#background. Accessed May 17, 2022.

22. The Jim Crow Period. Georgetown Law Library. Civil rights in the United States, a brief history: 1870s - 1950s. Available at: https://guides.ll.georgetown.edu/c.php?g=592919&p=4172697. Accessed May 17, 2022.

23. Novick L. Community Segregation, Redlining, and Public Health. J Public Health Manag Pract 2021; 27(5):435–6.

24. Krehbiel, Randy. Tulsa 1921 : Reporting a Massacre, University of Oklahoma Press, 2019. ProQuest Ebook Central.

25. Tulsa Race Riot. A report by the Oklahoma Commission to Study the Tulsa race riot of 1921. 2001. https://www.okhistory.org/research/forms/freport.pdf. [Accessed 25 July 2022].

26. Churchwell K, Elkind MSV, Benjamin RM, et al. Call to Action: Structural Racism as a Fundamental Driver of Health Disparities. Circulation 2020;142:e454–68.

27. Brands HW. Andrew Jackson: his life and times. New York: Anchor Books; 2006.

28. Britannica. Five Civilized Tribes. Encyclopedia Britannica. 2019. Available at: https://www.britannica.com/topic/Five-Civilized-Tribes. Accessed April, 2022.

29. Perdue T. The Legacy of Indian Removal. J South Hist 2012;78(1):3–36.

30. History.com. Trail of Tears. A&E Television Networks History Web site. 2009. Available at: https://www.history.com/topics/native-american-history/trail-of-tears. Accessed July 2020.

31. Manifest Destiny and Indian Removal. Smithsonian American Art Museum. Available at: https://americanexperience.si.edu/wp-content/uploads/2015/02/Manifest-Destiny-and-Indian-Removal.pdf. Accessed April, 2022.

32. President Andrew Jackson's Message to Congress "On Indian Removal"; 12/16/1830; Presidential Messages, 1789 - 1875; Records of the U.S. Senate,. Available at: https://www.archives.gov/milestone-documents/jacksons-message-to-congress-on-indian-removal. Accessed April, 2022.

33. Pauls EP. Trail of Tears. Encyclopedia Britannica Web site. 2021. Available at: https://www.britannica.com/event/Trail-of-Tears. Accessed May 17, 2022.

34. Bastrop PR. Episodes from the Genocide of the Native Americans: A Review Essay. Genocide Stud Prev An Int J 2007;2(2). Article 7.

35. Cameron SC, Phan LT. Ten stages of american indian genocide. Revista Interamericana de Psicologia/Interamerican J Psychol 2018;52(1):25–44.

36. National Academies of Sciences E, and Medicine; Health and Medicine Division; Board on Population Health and Public Health Practice; Committee on Community-Based Solutions to Promote Health Equity in the United States. In: Baciu A, Negussie Y, Geller A, et al, editors. Communities in action: Pathways to health equity. Washington (DC): National Academies Press (US); 2017. Appendix A, Native American Health: Historical and Legal Context. Available at: https://www.ncbi.nlm.nih.gov/books/NBK425854/.

37. Keating J. The Assimilation, Removal, and Elimination ofNative Americans. 2020. Available at: https://mcgrath.nd.edu/assets/390540/expert_guide_on_the_assimilation_removal_and_elimination_of_native_americans.pdf.

38. Hastings E. No longer a silent victim of history:" repurposing the documents of Japanese American internment. Arch Sci 2011;11(1–2):25–46.

39. Short History of Amache Japanese Internment Camp. Colorado state archives. Available at: https://archives.colorado.gov/sites/archives/files/Short%20History%20of%20Amache%20Japanese%20Internment%20Camp_0.pdf. Accessed May 18, 2022.

40. Gomez L. Manifest Destiny's Legacy: Race in America at the Turn of the Twentieth Century. 2007:117-147.

41. Yung J, Chang G, Lai H. Chinese American Voices : From the Gold Rush to the Present. In: University of California Press. 2006. Available at: http://ebookcentral.proquest.com/lib/howard/detail.action?docID=254866.

42. Lew-Williams B. The Chinese Must Go: Violence, Exclusion, and the Making of the Alien in America. In: Harvard University Press. 2018. Available at: http://www.jstor.org.proxyhu.wrlc.org/stable/j.ctv24trbsz.

43. Chinese exclusion act. History.com. 2018. Available at: https://www.history.com/topics/immigration/chinese-exclusion-act-1882. Accessed May 17, 2022.

44. Zesch S. Chinese Los Angeles in 1870-1871: The Makings of a Massacre. South Calif Q 2008;90(2): 109–58.

45. Chinese Immigration and the Chinese Exclusion Acts. US Department of State. Available at: https://history.state.gov/milestones/1866-1898/chinese-immigration#:~:text=In%201888%2C%20Congress%20took%20exclusion,unable%20to%20prevent%20its%20passage. Accessed May 17, 2022.

46. Burton JF, Farrell MM, Lord FB, et al. Confinement and Ethnicity: An Overview of World War II Japanese American Relocation Sites 2003;104(1):131–2.

47. Scherini RD. Executive Order 9066 and Italian Americans: The San Francisco Story. Calif Hist (San Francisco) 1991;70(4):366–77.

48. Halperin EC. The Jewish problem in U.S. medical education, 1920-1955. J Hist Med Allied Sci 2001; 56(2):140–67.

49. Halperin EC. Why Did the United States Medical School Admissions Quota for Jews End? Am J Med Sci 2019;358(5):317–25.

50. Kutner M, Greenberg E, Jin Y, et al. The Health Literacy of America's Adults: Results From the 2003 National Assessment of Adult Literacy (NCES 2006–483). Washington, DC: U.S. Department of Education; 2006.

51. Jackson K, Johnson RC, Persico C. The Effects of School Spending on Educational and Economic Outcomes: Evidence from School Finance Reforms. Q J Econ 2016;131(1):157–218.

52. Tackett KJ, Jenkins F, Morrell DS, et al. Structural racism and its influence on the severity of atopic dermatitis in African American children. Pediatr Dermatol 2020;37(1):142–6.

53. Creadore A, Desai S, Li SJ, et al. Insurance Acceptance, Appointment Wait Time, and Dermatologist Access Across Practice Types in the US. JAMA Dermatol 2021;157(2):181–8.

54. Adamson AS, Zhou L, Baggett CD, et al. Association of Delays in Surgery for Melanoma With Insurance Type. JAMA Dermatol 2017;153(11):1106–13.

55. Feng H, Berk-Krauss J, Feng PW, et al. Comparison of Dermatologist Density Between Urban and Rural Counties in the United States. JAMA Dermatol 2018;154(11):1265–71.

56. O'Reilly K. AMA: Racism is a threat to public health. American Medical Association Health Equity Web site. 2020. Available at: https://www.ama-assn.org/delivering-care/health-equity/ama-racism-threat-public-health. Accessed May 17, 2022.

Exploring Race, Racism, and Structural Racism in Medicine

Pamela S. Allen, MD[a],*, Natasha M. Mickel, PhD[b]

KEYWORDS

- Race • Racism • Structural racism • White privilege • Health disparities

KEY POINTS

- There are no genetic differences between races.
- Race is a man-made construct not a biological attribute.
- Race and racism are rooted in the man-made belief that the color of a person's skin and ethnic variation determines a person's hierarchal rank in humanity.
- Structural racism has led to health disparities in black and brown communities and is a public health crisis.

INTRODUCTION

Race and racism are rooted in the man-made belief that people with similar physical traits and ancestry should be categorized into distinct and separate races despite a lack of biological and genetic evidence. In the United States, the color of a person's skin has been used to determine their hierarchal rank in society. Early scientific theories of polygenics supported and perpetuated slavery and the concept of white supremacy. Worldwide, people of color have been thought of and treated as inferior to whites of European origin, which consequently has led to pervasive structural racism. Structural racism has in turn led to health disparities in black and brown communities. This article will explore the concepts of race and its origins, racism, and structural racism. Historical views, theories, and scientific findings will be reviewed regarding race. A by-product of racism, white privilege, and its manifestations will be discussed as well as the role of the US government. Finally, we will explore opportunities for individuals and institutions to become change agents of structural racism and champions for equity and inclusivity.

Race: A Man-Made Construct

Race is defined as the division of humans into groups based on common physical traits among people of shared ancestry. Hacking poignantly questioned "why has there been such a pervasive tendency to apply the category of race and to regard people of different races as essentially different kinds of people?"[1] Research reveals that there are no genetic differences between races. In fact, new findings in genetics debunk the theory. Geneticist Richard Lewontin examined the variation of protein in blood types. He grouped humans into 7 racial categories finding only 15% of protein in human blood varied across individuals. Thus, his data established no differences significant enough to support the concept of biological race.[2]

Rosenberg and colleagues[3] examined human diversity by studying 1056 subjects from 52 populations around the world using genotypes at 377 autosomal microsatellite loci. About 95% of genetic variance occurred in individuals within

[a] Department of Dermatology, University of Oklahoma College of Medicine, 619 Northeast 13th Street, Oklahoma City, OK 73104, USA; [b] Department of Family and Preventive Medicine, University of Oklahoma College of Medicine, Office of Diversity, Inclusion, and Community Engagement, 1105 North Stonewall Avenue, Oklahoma City, OK 73104, USA
* Corresponding author.
E-mail address: pamela-allen@ouhsc.edu

Dermatol Clin 41 (2023) 345–350
https://doi.org/10.1016/j.det.2022.08.005
0733-8635/23/Published by Elsevier Inc.

population. Only about 5% genetic variance was found between major groups. These findings support the fact that most human DNA is shared throughout different regions of the world. In the United States, race is primarily based on skin color and ethnic variation. Jablonski and Chaplin[4] applied the evolutionary theory that equatorial populations gradually developed dark skin, presumably to protect against ultraviolet radiation; whereas, people in northern latitudes developed pale skin to produce vitamin D from sunlight.

The reality is that socially defined racial groups in the United States, and throughout the world, differ in health outcomes. This is due to multiple factors including systemic differences in lived experience, social determinants of health and systemic racism, not genetics.[5] Ideally, we must strive to ensure that people of all races receive the same excellent health care.

RACE AND POLYGENETIC ORIGIN OF INFERIORITY

In the United States, there is a long history of racism and supporting racial theories that date to the eighteenth century. Monogenic theory purported that different races of men evolved from one ancestor. Polygenic theory surmised that each race had its own separate ancestral line or history. Both theories circulated throughout the United States during the late eighteenth century as colonialism advanced.[6] At that time one idea was widely accepted—that people of darker skin tones were fundamentally distinct from people with white skin, were inferior and should therefore, be treated differently. Both monogenic and polygenic theories supported the concept of Black inferiority and institution of slavery.[6]

During the turn of the nineteenth century, an American craniologist, Samuel Morton, researched racial differences in intelligence based on the size of human skulls and brains.[6,7] He concluded that Caucasians had the largest brain, thus proving to be the most intelligent, and Africans had the smallest brain inferring inferiority and lower intelligence. Morton believed he used scientific research to prove that Caucasians were intellectually superior compared with other races. In actuality, Morton and colleagues used a polygenetic origin of inferiority to maintain political control and societal hierarchy that promoted slavery.[6,7] This was the birth of scientific racism.

Josiah C. Nott, a Southern physician and slave owner, further supported and promoted the idea of polygenetics and race. In his 1850 essay entitled, "Essay on the Natural History of Mankind: Viewed in Connection with Negro Slavery," Nott argued that white, black, red, and yellow races came from distinct and different origins, which determined varying physical characteristics and intellectual abilities.[8] He rejected the scientific basis of Biblical creation theory, which states that mankind was divinely made from a single origin. Nott also attacked the theory of evolution stating that climate and lifestyle changes have limited effects on racial groups, "...they do not transform into another race but are fixed in that race typing at birth."[6,8] He believed that God "stamped the Negro Race with permanent inferiority" and that slavery was their natural place in society.[8]

Anthropologist Charles Darwin was dedicated to a monogenic, rather than a polygenic, view of human origins. However, he still divided humans and communities into distinct races according to differences in skin, eye, or hair color.[9] Darwin was convinced that evolution was advanced, and that the white race, particularly of European decent, were more advanced than the Black race, thus perpetuating race differences and racial hierarchy.[6,9]

Hogarth demonstrated how physicians during the late eighteenth century "medicalized" the Black race to determine disease susceptibility.[10] In the study of yellow fever in the Caribbean, Whites who had not adapted to the region seemed to be more devastated by the disease, whereas Blacks had little to no illness, seemingly due to natural immunity. This finding led to the popular belief that the bodies of Blacks experienced less physical suffering. This view not only defended Black slave labor in the Americas but rationalized the belief of race plurality. When Blacks did contract yellow fever, the physicians were unwilling to rethink race as a factor.[10]

As one explores historical racism, it is critically important to confront past mistakes and misunderstandings and strive to achieving a more fair and just society. Once accomplished, we can build on commonalities rather than differences.

WHITE PRIVILEGE: A CULTURAL NORMATIVE

Deeply rooted in European colonialism and the Atlantic slave trade, white privilege was established to preserve economic and political superiority and power over the Black population.[11] The term "white privilege" or "white skin privilege" refers to the receipt of unmerited societal benefits by someone who is white over someone who is nonwhite.[12]

White privilege does not equal racism. Rather it is the by-product of discriminatory acts of racism by an individual, group, or system with power and resources.[12,13]

Antiracism activist and scholar, Dr Peggy McIntosh, published seminal essays of her personal accounts of unearned white privilege which include having no fear of police or of traffic stops; ability to shop without being followed; the ability to observe people of her race at meetings and in the media; and never being asked to speak for all people of her racial group, to name a few.[12,13] From the owning and dehumanization of African slaves in the Americas to the repressive laws, segregation and restrictions placed on African Americans, known as Jim Crow Laws, to the recent police killings of Black and brown people, many will argue that White privilege continues to exist in everyday life as a cultural normative in the United States.

Scholar and activist, Theodore W. Allen, stated the need for White Americans to reject their white skin privileges in order to truly have a government of the people and by the people.[14] Steps toward dismantling white privilege include recognizing and acknowledging white privilege including one's own; using one's privilege to initiate discussion of and to denounce racism, become an activist in the face of potential ridicule and consequences of losing privilege, and education regarding historical and current societal issues surrounding racism.[11,13]

THE IMPACT OF STRUCTURAL RACISM ON HEALTH CARE

US healthcare policy has been historically rooted in structural racism. Structural racism is defined as the totality of ways in which societies foster racial discrimination through mutually reinforcing systems of housing, education, employment, earnings, benefits, credit, media, health care, and criminal justice. These patterns and practices in turn reinforce discriminatory beliefs, values, and distribution of resources.[15–26]

Yearby identified structural racism as the root cause of social determinants of health that lead to racial health disparities.[27,28] Structural racism is supported and reinforced through laws, policies, and patterns deemed normative. Examples of structural racism include Jim Crow Laws that deemed Blacks separate but equal; Fair Labor Standards Act of 1938 which excluded low-wage earners from paid sick leave; Home Owners' Loan Corporation lending policies that deemed minorities as a loan risk and limited their ability to own property; and disproportionate incarceration of people of color, limiting freedom and employment opportunities.[29–31] These laws and policies had cascading effects impacting wages, health benefits, K-12 education, neighborhood pollution and crime, food deserts, and public transportation, to name just a few. Structural injustices cause health inequities (ie, obesity, hypercholesterolemia, hypertension, and higher cardiovascular disease (CVD) and stroke mortality in Black Americans) that determine life expectancy.[29,31,32]

BECOMING A CHANGE AGENT AGAINST STRUCTURAL RACISM

Becoming a change agent against structural racism will require efforts from all sectors of society. It will be a long process of education, reflection, and action. Suggested first steps may include the following:

- Recognize and acknowledge that structural racism exists.
- Seek education regarding historical events, racial traumas, and systemic structures that developed out of the belief of superior and inferior races.
- Listen to personal experiences of people of color who have encountered racism.
- Learn about social and environmental barriers that hinder patients from achieving health equity and about their communities.
- Be an active participant in change.
- Participate in bias-training role-play.
- Call out racism when witnessed.
- Become involved in health-care policy and advocacy.

Structural change must begin with academic leaders who set the tone and tenor through institutional policies and practices for cultural inclusivity. It is important for educational institutions to move beyond talking points and written statements. They must determine how to include minoritize population in the leadership structure to assist with change.

It is important for diversity, equity, and inclusion (DEI) to be fully integrated into the lived and work experience of every learner, trainee, provider, faculty, and staff member within an academic health-care institution and be synonymous with academic excellence. Diversity, in and of itself, is not enough. Solomon and colleagues discuss promoting a structural framework for teaching antiracism in medical education.[31] They applied 4 steps proposed by Dr Camara P. Jones and others: see, name, understand, and act. This antiracism framework is similar to the medical process of clinical reasoning, addressing medical error, quality improvement, and constant self-growth and development.[33] Institutional transparency and accountability through the creation of reporting systems for racism and discrimination will lead to an environment of trust, support, and desire to do better.

To understand the underlying causes of racism at an institutional level, it is necessary to become data driven. Within medical education, it is important to identify and track implicit bias in standardized tests as well as the increasing attrition rate of underrepresented in medicine academic faculty.[33] The final step toward antiracism requires action. Action steps may include changes in medical admissions and curricula, learning environment, and institutional culture.[34]

With the changing landscape of our nation's demographics, which is projected to become majority non-white by 2045,[35] the establishment of pathway programs for underrepresented in medicine students can serve to promote racial equity in medicine. Mentorship and the recruitment of junior faculty will assist in the development of diverse leaders and clinical dermatologists;[36] and promote increased patient satisfaction,[37] better physician–patient communication,[38] and the potential to improve health outcomes.[39]

SUMMARY

This article has explored the social construct of race, its origins, and the development of racism in the United States. Historical views, theories, and scientific findings regarding race bring to light longstanding injustices and structures that support and perpetuate racism. Structural racism has played a significant role in health care and has led to health disparities that are prevalent today among minoritized populations. The strategy of seeing, naming, understanding, and acting is offered to initiate change, support antiracism, and ultimately strengthen our healthcare system.

CLINICS CARE POINTS

- There is a lack of significant genetic evidence that supports the concept of race.
- There is evidence that white privilege continues to exist in everyday life in the US.
- US healthcare laws and policies are historically embedded in structural racism.
- Structural racism is the root cause of social determinants of health leading to health inequities that determine life expectancy.
- Mentorship and recruitment of diverse faculty leaders and clinicians will help to improve patient experiences and overall care.
- Utilizing the 4-step process of seeing, naming, understanding, and acting is an

inital change to dismantle structural racism in medical education, support antiracism, and strengthen our healthcare system.

DISCLOSURE

The authors, P.S. Allen and N.M. Mickel, have no relevant financial relationships or affiliations with commercial interests to disclose.

REFERENCES

1. Hacking I. Why race still matters. Daedalus 2005; 134(1):102–16.
2. Lewontin RC. The apportionment of human diversity. In: Evolutionary biology. New York: Springer; 1972. p. 381–98.
3. Rosenberg NA, Pritchard JK, Weber JL, et al. Genetic structure of human populations. Science 2002;298(5602):2381–5.
4. Jablonski NG, Chaplin G. The colours of humanity: the evolution of pigmentation in the human lineage. Philosophical Trans R Soc B: Biol Sci 2017; 372(1724):20160349.
5. Goodman AH. Why genes don't count (for racial differences in health). Am J Public Health 2000;90(11): 1699.
6. Smith R. Types of mankind: polygenism and scientific racism in the nineteenth century United States scientific community. Pittsburg State University Digital Commons. (2014) Electronic Thesis Collection. Available at: https://digitalcommons.pittstate. edu/etd/105. Accessed July 17, 2022.
7. Menand L. Morton, Agassiz, and the Origins of Scientific Racism in the United States. Journal of Blacks in Higher Education. 2001/2002. 111-113. Available at: https://www.jstor.org/stable/pdf/ 3134139.pdf. Accessed July 17, 2022.
8. Nott JC. An Essay on the Natural History of Mankind: Viewed in Connection with Negro Slavery: delivered before the Southern Rights Association, 14th December, 1850. https://archive.org/details/ essayonnaturalhi00nott/page/16/mode/2up? q=brain. [Accessed 17 July 2022].
9. Shields A, Bhatia S. Darwin on race, gender, and culture. Am Psychol 2009;64(2):111.
10. Hogarth RA. Medicalizing Blackness: making racial difference in the Atlantic world, 1780-1840. Chapel Hill, NC: UNC Press Books; 2017.
11. Collins C. What Is White Privilege, Really? Recognizing white privilege begins with truly understanding the term itself. Teaching Tolerance 2018;(60):39–41.
12. McIntosh P., White Privilege and Male Privilege: a personal account of coming to see correspondences through work in women's studies, 1988,

Working paper No. 189. Wellesley, MA: Wellesley Center for Research on Women.

13. McIntosh P. White privilege: unpacking the invisible Knapsack. Philadelphia, PA: Peace & Freedom; 1989. p. 10–2.

14. Allen TW. John Brown Commemoration Committee, 100 West 82., New York, 24, New York, "A Call to join with sponsors of this Call in a John Brown Memorial Pilgrimage to Harper's Ferry, West Virginia on Saturday, December 4, 1965, cited in Perry, Jeffrey B. (July 2010).

15. Bailey ZD, Krieger N, Agénor M, et al. Structural racism and health inequities in the USA: evidence and interventions. Lancet 2017;389(10077): 1453–63.

16. Yearby R, Clark B, Figueroa JF. Structural Racism In Historical And Modern US Health Care Policy. Health Aff 2022;41(2):187–94.

17. Yearby R. Structural racism and health disparities: reconfiguring the social determinants of health framework to include the root cause. J Law Med Ethics 2020;48(3):518–26.

18. Ko L. Reproductive Rights: Unwanted Sterilization and Eugenics Programs in the United States. In: Beyond The Films. 2016. Available at: https://www.pbs.org/independentlens/blog/unwanted-sterilization-and-eugenics-programs-in-the-united-states. Accessed April 30, 2022.

19. The Pill: The Puerto Rico Pill Trials. In: American Experience. Available at: https://www.pbs.org/wgbh/americanexperience/features/pill-puerto-rico-pill-trials. Accessed April 1, 2022.

20. 1976: Government Admits Unauthorized Sterilization of Indian Women. Native Voices. US National Library of Medicine. Available at: https://www.nlm.nih.gov/nativevoices/timeline/543.html. Accessed April 1, 2022.

21. Stern AM. Forced Sterilization policies in the US targeted minorities and those with disabilities – and lasted into the 21st century. Institute for Healthcare Policy & Innovation. University of Michigan. 2020. https://ihpi.umich.edu/news/forced-sterilization-policies-us-targeted-minorities-and-those-disabilities-and-lasted-21st. [Accessed 16 July 2022].

22. The U.S. Public Health Service Syphilis Study at Tuskegee. Available at: https://www.cdc.gov/tuskegee/timeline.htm. Accessed April 1, 2022.

23. Structural Racism is a Public Health Crisis: Impact on the Black Community. American Public Health Association, 2020. Available at: https://www.apha.org/policies-and-advocacy/public-health-policy-statements/policy-database/2021/01/13/structural-racism-is-a-public-health-crisis. Accessed April 20, 2022.

24. Reyes M. The Disproportional Impact of COVID-19 on African Americans. Health Hum Rights 2020; 22(2):299–307.

25. Homandberg LK, Fuller-Rowell TE, et al. Experiences of Discrimination and Urinary Catecholamine Concentrations: Longitudinal Associations in a College Student Sample. Ann Behav Med 2020; 54(11):843–52.

26. Laurencin CT, Walker JM. Racial Profiling is a Public Health and Health Disparities Issue. Published in final form. J Racial Ethn Health Disparities 2020 Jun;7(3):393–7.

27. Yearby R. Structural Racism: The Root Cause of the Social Determinants of Health. Bill of Health: Examining the intersection of health law, biotechnology, and bioethics. 2020 Sep. Available at: https://blog.petrieflom.law.harvard.edu/2020/09/22/structural-racism-social-determinant-of-health/. Accessed July 16, 2022.

28. Braveman PA, Arkin E, Proctor D, et al. Systemic and Structural Racism: Definitions, Examples, Health Damages, and Approaches to Dismantling. Health Aff 2022;41(2). Available at: https://www.healthaffairs.org/doi/10.1377/hlthaff.2021.0139.

29. Civil Rights in America: Racial Discrimination in Housing. National Park Service. U.S. Department of the Interior national Historic Landmarks Program. https://www.nps.gov/subjects/nationalhistoriclandmarks/upload/Civil_Rights_Housing_NHL_Theme_Study_revisedfinal.pdf. [Accessed 17 July 2022].

30. Churchwell K, Elkind MSV, Benjamin RM, et al. Call to Action: Structural Racism as a Fundamental Driver of Health Disparities: A Presidential Advisory From the American Heart Association. Circulation 2020;142(24):142.e4-8.

31. Burke M. Moving Beyond the Statements: The Need for Action to Address Structural Racism at Predominantly White. Institutions 2020;5:174–9.

32. Baciu A, Negussie Y, Geller A, et al. The Root Causes of Health Inequity. In: Communities in Action: Pathways to Health Equity.2017. https://www.ncbi.nlm.nih.gov/books/NBK425845/. [Accessed 16 July 2022].

33. Solomon SR, Atalay AJ, Osman NY. Diversity Is Not Enough: Advancing a Framework for Antiracism in Medical Education. Acad Med 2021;96(11):1513–7.

34. Diaz T, Navarro JR, Chen EH. An Institutional Approach to Fostering Inclusion and Addressing Racial Bias: Implications for Diversity in Academic Medicine. Reaching Learn Med 2019;32(1):110–6.

35. Frey WH. The US will become 'minority white' in 2045, Census projects. The Avenue - Brookings. 2018. Available at: https://www.brookings.edu/blog/the-avenue/2018/03/14/the-us-will-become-minority-

white-in-2045-census-projects/. Accessed May 1, 2022.

36. Shim RS. Dismantling Structural Racism in Academic Medicine: A Skeptical Optimism. Acad Med 2020;95(12):1793–5.

37. LaVeist TA, et al. Is Doctor-Patient Race Concordance Associated with Greater Satisfaction with Care? J Health Soc Behav 2002;43(3):296–306.

38. Shen MJ, et al. The Effects of Race and Racial Concordance on Patient-Physician Communication: A Systematic Review of the Literature. J Racial Ethnic Health Disparities 2018;5:117–40.

39. Pandya AG, Alexis AF, Berger TG, et al. Increasing racial and ethnic diversity in dermatology: A call to action. J Am Acad Dermatol 2015;74(3):584–7.

Racial and Ethnic Disparities in Research and Clinical Trials

Nicole C. Syder, BA, Nada Elbuluk, MD, MSc*

KEYWORDS

- Skin of color • Ethnic skin • Health disparities • Diversity • Dermatology • Research • Health equity
- Clinical trials

KEY POINTS

- Racial and ethnic minorities are underrepresented in clinical trials across medical specialties including dermatology.
- Racial and ethnic minorities, particularly Blacks, have a documented history of mistreatment and human experimentation without consent.
- Multiple well-recognized physicians credited with significant medical advancements have a history of unethical medical practices against Blacks and other marginalized minority groups.
- There is inadequate reporting and representation of racially and ethnically diverse participants in dermatologic clinical trials.
- Lack of education, mistrust, and language barriers are concerns that should be addressed in order to recruit and retain racial and ethnic minorities as participants in research studies including clinical trials.

INTRODUCTION

Racial and ethnic minorities are underrepresented in medical research and clinical trials at numbers significantly lower than their overall population in the United States. Racial and ethnic minorities are defined as individuals identifying as Black, Hispanic/Latinx, Asian, American Indian, Alaska Native, and Pacific Islander.[1] In 2011, it was found that only 5% and 1% of participants in all clinical trials across medical specialties were Black and Hispanic, respectively.[2] Across various US clinical trials registered in ClinicalTrials.gov, there has been underrepresentation of racial/ethnic minorities.[3] For example, Black, Hispanic/Latinx, American Indian or Alaska Native, and mixed race individuals have been found to be underrepresented in stem cell clinical trials.[4] Another study

of cardiometabolic drugs (2008–2017) revealed that women and minorities, primarily Black individuals, were underrepresented in cardiac trials.[5] Vaccine clinical trials have also highlighted a near absence of Black, Indigenous and People of Color (BIPOC) communities.[6] Dermatology clinical trials unfortunately have also exhibited this trend, with studies revealing a lack of diversity in trials associated with conditions such as alopecia areata, atopic dermatitis, and acne.[7,8]

Possible contributing factors underpinning underrepresentation of racial ethnic minorities in clinical trails across specialities were discussed in a study conducted by Niranjan and colleagues.[9] They assessed bias and stereotyping when recruiting minorities for oncology clinical trials and found that clinical professionals viewed recruitment efforts for minority participants to be

Funding sources: None.
Reprint requests: Nada Elbuluk.
Department of Dermatology, Keck School of Medicine, University of Southern California, 830 South Flower Street, Ste 100, Los Angeles, CA 90017, USA
* Corresponding author.
E-mail address: nada.elbuluk@med.usc.edu

Dermatol Clin 41 (2023) 351–358
https://doi.org/10.1016/j.det.2022.10.007
0733-8635/23/© 2022 Elsevier Inc. All rights reserved.

challenging. They did not view potential minority recruits as ideal candidates, noting concerns for protocol compliance. Providers were found to withhold opportunities from potential minority study participants. Furthermore, they had misperceptions that potential minority participants had low knowledge of cancer clinical trials and used language barriers as another excuse to not enroll minorities. They also thought that certain minority patients were perceived as having distinct temperaments, making these discussions more difficult.

In addition to underrepresentation in clinical trials, there is overall underreporting of data on race and ethnicity. A systematic review was conducted to assess the representation of minorities in clinical trials that found that minorities were underrepresented in the trials, and that they were also underreported in the trials.[10] Of the clinical trials analyzed, 70.4% had no report on the race/ethnicity of study participants. NIH funded trials were found to be more consistent in reporting demographic characteristics likely due to NIH-specific policies that have been in place for several decades. In 1993, the National Institutes of Health passed its Revitalization Act requiring that all clinical trials receiving NIH funding include women and minority representation. Geller and colleagues[11] conducted a study assessing compliance with these guidelines and found that a large percentage of studies were noncompliant. Of 69 studies, 18% did not offer a breakdown of study participants by racial and ethnic group and 87% provided no analysis by race/ethnicity. Additionally, 87% of these studies did not report on any of their outcomes by sex and women were largely underrepresented. These findings are a sobering reflection of current clinical trial representation, which shows a lack of consistent compliance to these policies.

As the US continues to diversify, it is necessary that participants in clinical research be reflective of the general population. In 2011, Blacks and Hispanics made up 12% and 16% of the general US population, respectively.[2]

Historical Treatment of Racial and Ethnic Minorities in Medical Research

It has been documented that a contributor to challenges in the recruitment of minority populations into clinical trials and research studies stems from a deeply engrained history of mistrust of the health-care system.[12] Much of this mistrust is rooted in historical injustices and experimentation without consent against these marginalized populations. Several examples of this experimentation will be discussed in greater detail in this section.

Dr J. Marion Sims

The history of Dr J. Marion Sims, called the "Father of Gynecology," may be one of the oldest documented examples of human experimentation without consent and abuse of medical practices. Dr Sims, a renowned surgeon in the 1800s, was credited with the development of treatments for vesicovaginal fistula and antiseptic technique.[13] He built his practice in Montgomery, Alabama, by treating and conducting research on enslaved women without anesthesia. He operated under the widely held racist belief that Blacks did not feel pain. In situations where enslaved women were unable to reproduce due to gynecologic issues, they were brought to Dr Sims and became his property until treatment was complete. According to Dr Sims, there was never a time when he could not operate and because of this freedom, he considered it the most memorable time of his life.[14] Of note, many of the early vesicovaginal fistula surgeries were unsuccessful. One enslaved woman underwent 30 surgeries by Dr Sims before he became more skilled at the procedure.[14] After this time, he transitioned to operating on White women under anesthesia.

The Tuskegee Syphilis study

The Tuskegee Syphilis study is another historic example of unethical medical practice involving the Black community.[15] This study is one of many that have contributed to Black individuals' feeling distrust of the US health-care system. In 1932, the US Public Health Service began an experiment in Mason County, Alabama, assessing the natural course of untreated syphilis in Black men.[15] The study consisted of 400 Black men with syphilis and 200 uninfected Black men serving as controls. Penicillin became available in the 1950s for treatment of syphilis but study participants were not offered therapy. Treatment was deliberately withheld from study participants to gain scientific clarity on the natural course of syphilis at the expense of the increased morbidity and mortality of these men. Notably, the men participated in the study under the impression that they would be receiving treatment of "bad blood." They were given medications such as mercurial ointment and inadequate doses of neoarsphenamine, both ineffective treatments for syphilis. The original plan was to continue the study for 6 months but the study continued for years until 1972 when it was paused by the Department of Health, Education, and Welfare. By this time, likely more than 100 participants had died of causes directly related to advanced syphilis.[15] A system charged with doing no harm and saving lives deliberately withheld life-saving treatment from these men, leading to the death of many. This history is a significant reason the Black community remains weary of the motives of the health-care system.

Henrietta Lacks

The history of Henrietta Lacks reflects another example of research involving a minority individual without consent. Mrs. Lacks was a 31-year-old Black woman who presented to Johns Hopkins Hospital's Gynecology Clinic in Baltimore, MD, with complaints of spotting in between periods in 1951.[16] Physical examination revealed a lesion on her cervix that was subsequently biopsied. Biopsy specimens were sent to the pathology laboratory as well as Dr George Gey's tissue culture laboratory. Mrs. Lacks had provided consent for surgery but did not provide consent for her tissue samples to be shared and distributed in any manner.

Mrs. Lacks was diagnosed with epidermoid carcinoma, a very aggressive adenocarcinoma of the cervix. She underwent radiation treatment that was unsuccessful in slowing the spread of the disease and she ultimately died a few months after her initial presentation.

After the tissue samples were shared with Dr Gey's laboratory, her cells were cultured and then mass-produced and distributed to other colleagues. They were used for research on the polio and other vaccines. They were ultimately named HeLa cells in commemoration of her first and last name.[17] However, it took many years for Henrietta Lacks to actually be credited for the use of her cells and the scientific contribution, which came from them. Today, descendants of Henrietta Lacks have been vocal about the widespread use of her cells in laboratories around the world despite the original lack of informed consent. The use of Henrietta Lacks tissue and cells has had significant influence on medical research bioethics.

Dr Albert Kligman

Dr Albert Kligman was a dermatologist credited with the discovery of tretinoin in the 1960s while working as a medical researcher in dermatology at the University of Pennsylvania.[18] Dr Kligman's research and testing of tretinoin as well as various chemicals occurred on incarcerated individuals at the Holmesburg prison without consent. Of note, two-thirds of the experiment participants were Black. In 1960, he also conducted an experiment to study dioxin, which was applied to the foreheads and backs of the incarcerated men.[18] In some instances, he chose to apply 486 times the recommended dosage, leaving these men with various chronic dermatologic issues. Years later, Dr Kligman was quoted as saying things were

"simpler" before informed consent was required. He said, "No one asked me what I was doing. It was a wonderful time."[18] Since this time, several former inmates have come forward with complaints of long-term effects from the experimentation. In 1990, the city of Philadelphia, Holmesburg prison, and the University of Pennsylvania were all sued by a former inmate who believes he developed leukemia because of experiments in the prison. The suit was settled outside of court without any admission of guilt from the university.[19]

Summary

The examples of mistreatment and injustice against marginalized groups serve to foster a deep sense of mistrust of the health-care system among individuals from those communities. In various studies looking at the perceptions of Blacks of clinical research, lack of trust was a consistent theme.[12] Not only do these groups tend to lack trust for the health-care system as a whole, the overall research process and the researchers themselves are often deemed untrustworthy.

In addition to this mistrust, additional common barriers to the participation of Blacks in clinical research include issues with communication, lack of awareness of research opportunities, logistics associated with the research, and type of study.[20] Studies have found that Blacks are willing to agree to participate in studies with low perceived risk, such as surveys or providing urine or blood samples.[21,22] They are less likely to agree to more perceived high-risk studies involving medications or injections. Logistical issues pertaining to the time commitment for participation, transportation, and childcare services have also been cited as a few additional barriers inhibiting the participation of Blacks in clinical trials.[23]

Racial and Ethnic Diversity in Dermatologic Research and Clinical Trials

Disparities in dermatologic clinical trials

Clinical trials allow for the approval of new drugs and therapies as well as provide important information on the safety and efficacy of novel treatments. Dermatology, similar to many other fields in medicine, currently lacks adequate representation of racial and ethnic minorities in clinical trials. There have been few studies conducted to evaluate this issue (Table 1). One study examined racial and ethnic diversity as well as reporting of minority groups in all randomized clinical trials (RCTs) related to alopecia areata, atopic dermatitis, acne, psoriasis, vitiligo, lichen planus, and seborrheic dermatitis conducted from 2010 to

Table 1
Racial and ethnic diversity data for dermatologic clinical trials

	Author, Year	White, % (N)	Black/African American, % (N)	Hispanic, % (N)	Asian, % (N)	American Indian or Alaskan Native, % (N)	Native Hawaiian/ Pacific Islander, % (N)	Mixed Race, % (N)	Other/ Unspecified, % (N)
Combined data for SOC studies[7,28]	Charrow et al,[7] 2017	72% (8016/11140)	13% (1446/11140)	14.7% (1639/11140)	3.3% (370/11140)	-	-	-	-
	Ferguson et al,[28] 2021[a]	72.9%	8.4%	5.3%	5.2%	0.13%	0.17%	-	7.8%
Clinical trials for dermatological drugs[25]	Ding et al, 2021	80.4% (28065/34890)	9.8% (3242/33240)	18.9% (2614/13860)	5.5% (1535/27696)	-	-	-	-
Acne[31]	Montgomery et al,[31] 2021	-	10.3% (34/330)	4.8% (16/330)	54.7% (181/330)	-	-	21.8% (72/330)	8.2% (27/330)
Acne- Pediatrics[34]	Ding et al, 2021	71.9% (20695/28771)	17.6% (5066/28771)	30.4% (6384/28771)	5.9% (1698/28771)	0.5% (136/28771)	0.3% (89/28771)	-	-
Atopic dermatitis[8,27,31]	Price et al,[8] 2020	54% (5301/9808)	8.9% (871/9808)	3.7% (365/9808)	16.2% (1585/9808)	0.2% (17/9808)	0.2% (20/9808)	20.5% (2014/9808)	20.5% (2014/9808)
	Montgomery et al,[31] 2021	-	17.1% (62/361)	2.2% (8/361)	63% (228/361)	-	-	11.3% (41/361)	6.1% (22/361)
	Hirano et al,[27] 2012	62.1% (13679/22202)	18% (3954/22202)	2% (441/22202)	6.9% (1523/22202)	0.02% (4/22202)	0.3% (57/22202)	0.05% (12/22202)	6.8% (1506/22202)
Dyschromia[31]	Montgomery et al,[31] 2021	-	8.2% (41/498)	9.6% (48/498)	64.1% (319/498)	-	-	11.1% (55/498)	7.0% (35/498)
Hidradenitis Suppurativa[33]	Price et al,[33] 2021	68% (669/984)	14% (138/984)	1.5% (15/984)	2.9% (29/984)	0.3% (3/984)	0.1% (1/984)	-	14.6% (144/984)
Psoriatic Arthritis and Biologic Treatments[24]	Shwe et al,[24] 2021	80.60% (6082/7500)	0.40% (30/7500)	6.19% 467/7500	3.56% (269/7500)	0.61% (46/7500)	0.08% (6/7500)	0.45% (34/7500)	8.11% (612/7500)

[a] N values were not provided for this study.

2015.[7] It found that merely 11.3% of international studies and 59.8% of US studies reported the racial/ethnic demographic characteristics of participants. Of the 59.8% of US studies with recorded race/ethnicity, 74.4% of these participants were White. Findings such as this highlight the lack of diversity in dermatologic clinical trials and the underreporting of demographic data.

A recent cross-sectional study sought to assess the representation of minorities in clinical trials using biologic agents for the treatment of psoriatic arthritis from 2020 to 2021. Only half of the studies reported race and ethnicity, 44% reported only race, and 6% reported only ethnicity.[24] Most participants were White (80.6%). The percentages of Black, Asian, American Indian, and Native Hawaiian/Pacific Islander participants were 0.40%, 3.56%, 0.61%, and 0.08%, respectively. Similar findings were seen in a study on clinical trials for drugs for dermatologic diseases. A total of 36 novel drugs approved by the Food and Drug Administration between 1995 and 2019 were assessed. White participants were overrepresented at 80.4%, with Black and Asian participants comprising 9.8% and 5.5%, respectively.[25]

Price and colleagues recently looked at disparities in clinical trials for atopic dermatitis. A total of 33 randomized clinical trials worldwide were included with 82% of the trials including information on the race and/or ethnicity of study participants.[8] Of these trials, 81% included race exclusively and 19% included both. More than 50% of participants across all studies were White (54%), whereas Asians and those who were Black and of African descent comprised 16.2% and 8.9% of participants, respectively. Despite the health disparities of Blacks with atopic dermatitis including Black children being 6 times more likely to develop severe atopic dermatitis than their White counterparts, there continue to be insufficient numbers of Blacks in atopic dermatitis clinical trials.[26] An earlier study similarly assessed reporting of diversity of clinical trials in atopic dermatitis (2000–2009) in the United States and found reporting rates of race and ethnicity to be 59.5% and that White participants were overrepresented across all included studies.[27] During the 9 years of the study, there continued to be no significant improvement in diversity numbers.

A systematic review identified all randomized clinical trials between 2005 and 2020 related to acne/acneiform eruptions, lichen planus, vitiligo, psoriasis, eczema, seborrheic dermatitis, vitiligo, atopic dermatitis, and alopecia areata.[28] A total of 287 US-based studies and 1217 non-US studies were included and trends in reporting and diversity of participants were recorded. During the 15-year period, there was an increase in the reporting of race/ethnicity. The percentage of Black participants decreased from 8.8% to 8.4%, American Indian participants increased from 0.11% to 0.13%, Pacific Islander decreased from 0.24% to 0.17% and Hispanic also decreased from 5.5% to 5.3%. Of note, Asian representation increased from 1.8% to 5.2%.

Chen and colleagues recently compared levels of racial/ethnic representation between dermatologic clinical trials conducted between 2010 to 2015 and 2015 to 2020. They found that in comparison to the period from 2010 to 2015, clinical trials from 2015 to 2020 had an increased rate of racial/ethnic reporting. However, the proportion of studies containing a percentage of racial/ethnic minorities representative of the US population remained unchanged at 38.1%. Additionally, psoriasis trials in particular were shown to be the least diverse.[29]

Research on conditions disproportionately affecting skin of color

The 3 most common dermatologic chief complaints for individuals with SOC are acne, dyschromia, and atopic dermatitis.[30] A study evaluated the quantity of peer-reviewed research on these conditions in SOC and found that only 1.6% of the studies were specific to SOC.[31] Of those studies, the majority of them were conducted in Asian populations with 54.7% representation in acne studies, 63% in atopic dermatitis, and 64.1% in dyschromias. The research included in this article was not exclusive to clinical trials and included all research conducted in SOC. Research studies focused on skin of color (SOC) are lacking in darker skin types, particularly Fitzpatrick skin type IV through VI.[31]

There are also limited trials on conditions that disproportionately affect SOC populations such as keloids, central centrifugal cicatricial alopecia, and hidradenitis suppurative. Hidradenitis suppurativa (HS), a debilitating, chronic disease with increased prevalence among Blacks has also been found to lack diversity in its trials.[32] One of few studies assessing the distribution of race/ethnicity in HS RCTs found that among the most recent trials from 2000 to 2019, 68% of participants were White and 14% were Black or African American.[33] Only 2.9%, 0.3%, and 0.1% were Asian, American Indian/Alaska native, and Native Hawaiian or Pacific Islander, respectively.

Pediatric dermatology

Interestingly, disparities in pediatric clinical trials in dermatology do not seem to mirror those of adult trials. Acne vulgaris is considered the most common skin disease and is highly prevalent among women and children.[34] Randomized clinical trials between 2006 and 2018 on pediatric acne treatment were assessed for the level of reporting and representation of race/ethnicity. The frequency of reporting of race/ethnicity was found to be relatively low. Race and ethnicity was reported in 61.3% and 46.8% of all RCTs, respectively.[34] White participants predominated, however, the proportions of various races were more representative of the general population. Black, Asian, and Hispanic/Latinx participants comprised 17.6%, 5.9%, and 30.4% of clinical trials, respectively.

Call to Action

Addressing the issue of insufficient racial/ethnic diversity and reporting in research and clinical trials will require a multiprong approach. For SOC communities, robust community engagement and relationship building are tools that have been found to be helpful in increasing participation in clinical trials.[6] A study looking at the recruitment and retention of Blacks in clinical trials found the most commonly used strategies included distribution of fliers at various community-based locations such as outpatient clinics and recreational centers, advertising in local newspapers that the population of interest was likely to read, speaking to patients at their regular clinic visits, field-based community outreach, and "snowballing" in which participants would tell friends and family about studies that were of interest to them. Notably, the most effective strategy was found to be the field-based approach in which researchers looking to recruit would go into the community and explain the study to potential participants. Newspaper advertisements and snowballing were the next most effective means of recruitment.[35]

Working with community-based and religious-based organizations, such as churches, is another grassroots strategy for increasing participation in research initiatives, particularly in the Black community.[36] Additional recommendations for increasing clinical trial diversity center largely around the education of minority communities on clinical trials. A significant barrier to low participation is lack of education on the purpose and implications of such research studies.[37] Community information sessions should be held and widely accessible to those interested in learning more. Additionally, language differences can also be a considerable barrier to participation. Bilingual and culturally diverse medical and research staff are incredibly helpful to address this issue and to help foster trust between potential participants and researchers.

Cultural competence also plays an important role in improving diversity in research.

This includes providing services that are respectful and considerate of the health beliefs, practices, cultural, and linguistic needs of diverse populations.[38] The lack of cultural competence among researchers and health-care providers has been indicated as a considerable barrier to the participation of minorities in research and contributes to feelings of mistrust.[39] When researchers exhibit cultural competency and respect for the cultural practice of their target population, they are more equipped to develop strategies for effective recruitment. Having a research team member of a similar identity can aid in community engagement efforts.[35]

Race concordant interactions are also helpful to establish rapport with minority individuals.[2] Coakley and colleagues suggests that increased representation of minority physicians is an important factor in increasing the number of minority patients open to participating in clinical trials. Additionally, Gorbatenko-Roth and colleagues[40]. conducted a cross-sectional study assessing Black patients' perceptions of their dermatologic care and found that, overall, patient–dermatologist racial concordance was preferred. This kind of rapport and trust, which has been shown to improve clinical care and health-care outcomes, can also help with increased study recruitment.

Beyond recruitment, it also critical to establish strategies for the retention of study participants. Intensive follow-up and communication have been found to improve participation as well as retention.[41] The importance of maintaining the same interviewers or research field staff has also been emphasized as a simple, yet impactful, means of encouraging participants to remain in research studies.

Stronks and colleagues made a compelling argument for diversity efforts that included more than just a blanket declaration to work to increase the inclusion of minorities in clinical trials. They proposed a more comprehensive and methodological strategy that includes designing entirely new RCTs that test specific treatments that have already been studied in trials comprising more homogenous groups.[42] Another proposed option is to increase the allotment of participants in ongoing clinical trials, thus creating an opportunity to increase the representation of minorities within these studies.

SUMMARY

Diverse and equitable representation in clinical research is essential for the development of safe and efficacious therapies for all patients. Oh and colleagues[43] discusses the importance of diversity in clinical trials citing that adequate representation of various racial/ethnic groups grants us the opportunity to study the impact of ancestral influences, social factors, and environmental exposures on health outcomes. Knowing that disease patterns and clinical responses to treatment can vary significantly by racial and ethnic background, it is prudent that research studies include diverse populations.[43]

Diverse representation of minority groups in clinical trials is necessary so that the results can be made generalizable to various demographic groups including minority populations.[44] Expanding the representation of these populations in medical research including clinical trials continues to be an important and significant challenge.

Recent data support the persistence of inadequate representation of racial/ethnic minority groups within dermatology. This limitation can contribute to health disparities and result in further widening of the gap in health outcomes between SOC individuals and their White counterparts. Policies such as those created by NIH-funded trials requiring adequate representation of minorities are necessary to increase adherence to reporting and diversifying pools of participants. There have been important strides and policies created to improve the current underrepresentation of racial and ethnic minorities in research but significant work remains. Dermatology as a specialty must recognize these gaps and work toward making participation in dermatologic research including clinical trials more representative of our continually diversifying nation.

CONFLICTS OF INTEREST

Dr N. Elbuluk is the director of the USC Dermatology Diversity and Inclusion Program as well as the Director of the Skin of Color and Pigmentary Disorders Program at the USC Department of Dermatology, Keck School of Medicine.

REFERENCES

1. America's Racial and Ethnic Minorities. PRB. Available at: https://www.prb.org/resources/americas-racial-and-ethnic-minorities/. Accessed December 14, 2021.
2. Coakley M, Fadiran EO, Parrish LJ, et al. Dialogues on diversifying clinical trials: successful strategies for engaging women and minorities in clinical trials. J Womens Health 2002 2012;21(7):713–6.
3. Turner BE, Steinberg JR, Weeks BT, et al. Race/ethnicity reporting and representation in US clinical trials: a cohort study. Lancet Reg Health – Am 2022; 0(0). https://doi.org/10.1016/j.lana.2022.100252.
4. Parvanova I, Finkelstein J. Disparities in Racial and Ethnic Representation in Stem Cell Clinical Trials. Importance Health Inform Public Health Pandemic 2020;358–61. https://doi.org/10.3233/SHTI200569.
5. Khan MS, Shahid I, Siddiqi TJ, et al. Ten-year trends in enrollment of women and minorities in pivotal trials supporting recent us food and drug administration approval of novel cardiometabolic drugs. J Am Heart Assoc 2020;9(11). https://doi.org/10.1161/JAHA.119.015594.
6. Andrasik MP, Broder GB, Wallace SE, et al. Increasing Black, Indigenous and People of Color participation in clinical trials through community engagement and recruitment goal establishment. PLoS ONE 2021;16(10):e0258858.
7. Charrow A, Xia FD, Joyce C, et al. Diversity in dermatology clinical trials: a systematic review. JAMA Dermatol 2017;153(2):193–8.
8. Price KN, Krase JM, Loh TY, et al. Racial and ethnic disparities in global atopic dermatitis clinical trials. Br J Dermatol 2020;183(2):378–80.
9. Niranjan SJ, Martin MY, Fouad MN, et al. Bias and stereotyping among research and clinical professionals: Perspectives on minority recruitment for oncology clinical trials. Cancer 2020;126(9):1958–68.
10. Rochon PA, Mashari A, Cohen A, et al. The inclusion of minority groups in clinical trials: problems of under representation and under reporting of data. Account Res 2004;11(3–4):215–23.
11. Geller SE, Adams MG, Carnes M. Adherence to federal guidelines for reporting of sex and race/ethnicity in clinical trials. J Womens Health 2002 2006;15(10):1123–31.
12. Luebbert R, Perez A. Barriers to clinical research participation among African Americans. J Transcult Nurs 2016;27(5):456–63.
13. Sartin JS, Sims JM. the father of gynecology: hero or villain? South Med J 2004;97(5):500–5.
14. Holland B. The 'father of modern gynecology' performed shocking experiments on enslaved women. HISTORY. Available at: https://www.history.com/news/the-father-of-modern-gynecology-performed-shocking-experiments-on-slaves. Accessed December 10, 2021.
15. Brandt AM. Racism and research: the case of the tuskegee syphilis study. Hastings Cent Rep 1978; 8(6):21–9.
16. Sodeke SO, Powell LR. Paying tribute to henrietta lacks at tuskegee university and at the virginia henrietta lacks commission, richmond, virginia. J Health Care Poor Underserved 2019;30(4S):1–11.
17. McGehee Harvey A. Johns Hopkins–the birthplace of tissue culture: the story of Ross G. Harrison, Warren H. Lewis and George O. Gey. Johns Hopkins Med J 1975;136(3):142–9.

18. Lasting Scars: Albert Kligman and the Holmesburg Prison Experiments. Available at: https://projects.34st.com/2021/street-features/. Accessed December 7, 2021.

19. U. involved in chemical tests on prisoners | The Daily Pennsylvanian. Available at: https://www.thedp.com/article/1995/05/u-involved-in-chemical-tests-on-prisoners. Accessed April 7, 2022.

20. Owens OL, Jackson DD, Thomas TL, et al. African American men's and women's perceptions of clinical trials research: focusing on prostate cancer among a high-risk population in the South. J Health Care Poor Underserved 2013;24(4):1784–800.

21. Freimuth VS, Quinn SC, Thomas SB, et al. African Americans' views on research and the Tuskegee Syphilis Study. Soc Sci Med 1982 2001;52(5):797–808.

22. Slomka J, Ratliff EA, McCurdy S, et al. Perceptions of risk in research participation among underserved minority drug users. Subst Use Misuse 2008;43(11):1640–52.

23. Brown RF, Cadet DL, Houlihan RH, et al. Perceptions of participation in a phase I, II, or III clinical trial among African American patients with cancer: what do refusers say? J Oncol Pract 2013;9(6):287–93.

24. Shwe S, Nguyen C, Bhutani T. Racial disparities in clinical trials of biologic treatments for psoriatic arthritis. J Am Acad Dermatol 2021. https://doi.org/10.1016/j.jaad.2021.08.038. S0190-9622(21)02381-1.

25. Ding J, Zhou Y, Khan MS, et al. Representation of sex, race, and ethnicity in pivotal clinical trials for dermatological drugs. Int J Womens Dermatol 2021;7(4):428–34.

26. Poladian K, De Souza B, McMichael AJ. Atopic dermatitis in adolescents with skin of color. Cutis 2019;104(3):164–8.

27. Hirano SA, Murray SB, Harvey VM. Reporting, representation, and subgroup analysis of race and ethnicity in published clinical trials of atopic dermatitis in the United States between 2000 and 2009. Pediatr Dermatol 2012;29(6):749–55.

28. Ferguson JE, Vetos D, Ho BV, et al. Trends in diversity of participants in dermatology clinical trials over time: a systematic review. J Am Acad Dermatol 2021. https://doi.org/10.1016/j.jaad.2021.05.052. S0190-9622(21)01090-2.

29. Chen V, Akhtar S, Zheng C, et al. Assessment of Changes in Diversity in Dermatology Clinical Trials Between 2010-2015 and 2015-2020: A Systematic Review. JAMA Dermatol 2022. https://doi.org/10.1001/jamadermatol.2021.5596.

30. Alexis AF, Sergay AB, Taylor SC. Common dermatologic disorders in skin of color: a comparative practice survey. Cutis 2007;80(5):387–94.

31. Montgomery SNB, Elbuluk N. A quantitative analysis of research publications focused on the top chief complaints in patients with skin of color. J Am Acad Dermatol 2021;85(1):241–2.

32. Vlassova N, Kuhn D, Okoye G. Hidradenitis suppurativa disproportionately affects African Americans: a single-center retrospective analysis. Acta Derm Venereol 2015;95(8):990–1.

33. Price KN, Hsiao JL, Shi VY. Race and ethnicity gaps in global hidradenitis suppurativa clinical trials. Dermatol Basel Switz 2021;237(1):97–102.

34. Ding J, Haq AF, Joseph M, et al. Disparities in pediatric clinical trials for acne vulgaris: A cross-sectional study. J Am Acad Dermatol 2021. https://doi.org/10.1016/j.jaad.2021.10.013. S0190-9622(21)02654-2.

35. Otado J, Kwagyan J, Edwards D, et al. Culturally competent strategies for recruitment and retention of African American populations into clinical trials. Clin Transl Sci 2015;8(5):460–6.

36. Yancey AK, Ortega AN, Kumanyika SK. Effective recruitment and retention of minority research participants. Annu Rev Public Health 2006;27:1–28.

37. Kailas A, Dawkins M, Taylor SC. Suggestions for increasing diversity in clinical trials. JAMA Dermatol 2017;153(7):727.

38. Taylor SC, Heath C. Cultural competence and unique concerns in patients with ethnic skin. J Drugs Dermatol JDD 2012;11(4):460–5.

39. Chalela P, Suarez L, Muñoz E, et al. Promoting factors and barriers to participation in early phase clinical trials: patients perspectives. J Community Med Health Educ 2014;4(281):1000281.

40. Gorbatenko-Roth K, Prose N, Kundu RV, et al. Assessment of black patients' perception of their dermatology care. JAMA Dermatol 2019;155(10):1129–34.

41. Russell C, Palmer JR, Adams-Campbell LL, et al. Follow-up of a large cohort of Black women. Am J Epidemiol 2001;154(9):845–53.

42. Stronks K, Wieringa NF, Hardon A. Confronting diversity in the production of clinical evidence goes beyond merely including under-represented groups in clinical trials. Trials 2013;14:177.

43. Oh SS, Galanter J, Thakur N, et al. Diversity in clinical and biomedical research: a promise yet to be fulfilled. PLoS Med 2015;12(12):e1001918.

44. Burchard EG, Ziv E, Coyle N, et al. The importance of race and ethnic background in biomedical research and clinical practice. N Engl J Med 2003;348(12):1170–5.

Diversity, Equity, and Inclusion Initiatives in Dermatology Organizations

Ananya Munjal, MS[a], Nkanyezi Ferguson, MD[b],*

KEYWORDS

- Diversity, equity, and inclusion • Underrepresented in medicine
- American Academy of Dermatology

KEY POINTS

- Over the past several years, there has been an active effort to incorporate Diversity, Equity, and Inclusion (DEI) initiatives in US dermatologic societies.
- Ongoing DEI initiatives in US dermatology organizations include establishment of DEI committees, creation and distribution of educational resources, increased mentorship for dermatology trainees who are underrepresented in medicine (URiM), and establishment of funding for skin of color research.
- It is imperative that we work towards strengthening DEI programs supporting URiM trainees in an effort to create systemic change in the field of dermatology.

INTRODUCTION

Throughout the course of the past several years, the COVID-19 pandemic and subsequent racial justice movements have highlighted racial and ethnic heath care inequities that persist in our society. Dermatology is one of the least diverse medical specialties, and the current demographic of dermatology providers in the United States is unrepresentative of the population—although black and Hispanic people make up a combined 31% of the US population, they only represent 7.2% of dermatology providers.[1,2]

It is crucial that health care providers reflect the growing diversification of the United States, as it is predicted that minority groups will comprise greater than 50% of the American population by 2044.[3] Diversity, Equity, and Inclusion (DEI) initiatives play a critical role in creating systemic change and disassembling racial health disparities in the institutions responsible for our health and well-being. Here, the authors detail the ongoing efforts and DEI initiatives being undertaken by US dermatologic societies in an effort to provide the best possible care for people of all backgrounds and create a health care landscape more reflective of the patients served (**Table 1**).

AMERICAN ACADEMY OF DERMATOLOGY
American Academy of Dermatology Diversity Committee

The American Academy of Dermatology (AAD) Diversity Committee established a 3-year (2021–2023) DEI plan, approved by the AAD Board of Directors, to further the Academy's strategic goal of increasing access to dermatologic care through fostering diversity in the dermatology specialty and increasing dermatologic services available to underserved populations.[4] This four-pronged plan was developed to (1) Promote and facilitate DEI within AAD governance and programs, (2) Ensure education and research encompass health disparities and skin of color and advocate for black

The authors do not have any commercial or financial conflicts of interest and have not received funding for this project.
[a] University of Iowa Carver College of Medicine, 375 Newton Road, Iowa City, IA 52242, USA; [b] Department of Dermatology, University of Missouri, 1020 Hitt Street, Columbia, MO 65212, USA
* Corresponding author.
E-mail address: nkanyezi-ferguson@uiowa.edu

Dermatol Clin 41 (2023) 359–369
https://doi.org/10.1016/j.det.2022.10.008

Table 1
Themes in diversity, equity, and inclusion initiatives across dermatology organizations

Theme	Goal	Examples/Programs
Organization-specific DEI Committees	Institution of DEI committees to focus efforts on expanding access	• AAD Diversity Committee • APD DEI workgroup • SID Diversity and Inclusion committee • ASDS Diversity, Equity, and Inclusion Work Group • SPD Equity, Diversity, and Inclusion committee • SOCS Diversity in Action Task Force • WDS Diversity, Equity, and Inclusion Committee
Statements against racial inequality and prompting DEI missions	To publicly denounce racism and other forms of discrimination and detail ongoing DEI initiatives	• Example from AAD: "Interventions to eliminate health disparities must be comprehensive and integrated into the education of FAAD dermatologists" • Example from APD: "[We] stand strongly in support of our colleagues in residency and fellowship leadership as well as our trainees who come from diverse backgrounds, especially those from groups historically marginalized in our country." • Example from SOCS: "The Skin of Color Society strongly denounces prejudice, discrimination and violence in all of its forms, directed at any and all individuals and groups." • Example from ASDS: ASDS position statement opposing all forms of bias and discrimination • Example from SPD: "The SPD Committee on EDI supports all communities targeted by violence and discrimination and remains invested in anti-bigotry." • Example from WDS: "The mission of the Women's Dermatologic Society DEI Committee is to cultivate diversity, equity, and inclusion within dermatology through the creation of educational experiences, scholarly opportunities, and collegial support." • Example from NMA Derm: editorial: "A Time for Resolve, Change, Unity, and Hope"
Medical student initiatives	To increase representation of URiM medical students in dermatology	• WDS Summer Research Fellowship • AAD/A Pathways: Inclusivity in Dermatology Program • SNMA Medical Student Mentoring • APD/NMA Derm Mentorship Program • NMA Derm Mentorship Program • SOCS Mentorship Program • ASDS Rise Up Mentorship Program
Residency-focused initiatives	To increase representation of URiM applicants selected for dermatology residency	• AAD/A Pathways: Inclusivity in Dermatology Program • Diversity Champion Workshop hosted in collaboration with AAD, APD, and SID

(*continued on next page*)

Theme	Goal	Examples/Programs
		<ul><li>SOCS Observership Grant, Mentorship Program, and Dermatology Residency Application Process Town Hall</li><li>APD Promotion of increased diversity in dermatology resident recruitment</li><li>SPD Underrepresented in Medicine Mentorship Award for residents</li><li>WDS UIM Resident Mentorship Award</li></ul>
Outside resource links	To promote the accessibility of information on patients with skin of color	<ul><li>AAD Diversity Committee Information Report</li><li>ASDS link to AMA STEPS Forward Toolkit "Racial and Health Equity: Concrete STEPS for Health Systems"</li><li>SID link to "Diversity and Inclusion Toolkit" resource page with DEI-suggested readings</li><li>SOCS linked resources to skin of color textbooks and list of ethnic skin centers</li><li>SPD links to antiracist resources, readings, toolkits, and support groups, and publishing of diversity-focused patient perspectives handouts</li></ul>
Research	To support dermatology research by URiM students and increase funding for skin of color research	<ul><li>AAD A. Paul Kelly, MD Research Award</li><li>SID Freinkel Diversity Fellows Program</li><li>WDS Summer Research Fellowship for URiM students</li><li>SOCS Research Award, Career Development Award, and Grant Writing Webinar to promote dermatology research within the field of skin of color</li><li>SPD Special Issue of Pediatric Dermatology Equity, Diversity, & Inclusion</li><li>NMA Derm John A. Kenney Resident and Fellow Research Symposium</li></ul>

Table 1 *(continued)*

and Latino patient representation in research, (3) Expand the Academy's advocacy priorities to include addressing health inequities and increase the number of underrepresented in medicine (URiM) dermatologists, and (4) Provide leadership and professional development programming.[5]

To date, this 3-year plan has increased the percentage of URiM committee, council, and task force appointments, significantly increased the amount of virtual meeting experience diversity content from 2020 to 2021, established 2 new named awards and lectureships, encouraged increased minority representation in the Journal of the American Academy of Dermatology editorial board and authorship, and supported access and funding for telehealth in underserved areas. The committee is now working toward reviewing the selection process for all members of dermatology leadership programs, improving public availability of skin of color images, increasing skin of color curriculum, developing programs for URiM faculty and trainees, improving education on health disparities, and establishing a Leadership Institute conference for URiM residents.

Although the Academy initiatives are primarily patient and member focused, there are additional initiatives to enhance staff Human Resource processes to optimize access, hiring, and talent development. Cultural immersion programs have been established to enhance awareness and understanding to foster diverse talent and elevate voices across the company.

In 2021, the AAD published a formal "Position Statement on Dermatology Workforce Diversity and Health Disparities" that details the importance of understanding the underlying cause of health disparities. This position statement acknowledges the need for elevating physician awareness of social determinants of health and health disparities; improving access to care for marginalized patients and communities; ensuring that research, scholarships, and publications promote health equity; diversifying the dermatologist workforce and organizational leadership; and supporting policies addressing institutional inequities outside of health care that lead to poor health outcomes.[6]

In recognition of the need to collaborate and coordinate efforts across the dermatology specialty as a whole, an Intersociety Diversity Workgroup was created, which was later formally transitioned to a sustainable Task Force. The primary purpose of the AAD Intersociety Diversity Task Force is to "support the goals and facilitate awareness, communication, and implementation of the AAD Diversity, Equity, and Inclusion initiatives. This is achieved by coordinating efforts across dermatologic societies to maximize expertise, organization strengths and infrastructure. The Task Force is designed to identify shared goals and roles, as well as define and clarify joint opportunities and industry partnerships that help to meet and accomplish mission, goals, resources, and funding." The task force now includes the dermatologic societies AAD, Association of Professors of Dermatology (APD), Skin of Color Society (SOCS), Society for Investigative Dermatology (SID), Women's Dermatology Society (WDS), National Medical Association (NMA) Dermatology Section, and American Society of Dermatologic Surgeons (ASDS) and has collaborated with the National Hispanic Association, and the program, Nth Dimensions.

In 2019, the task force founded the Diversity Champion Workshop with a focus on inclusion, recruiting minority trainees, and better serving underserved patient populations. The workshop was designed for faculty members in dermatology residency programs involved in the evaluation and selection of residency candidates. Through this initiative, dermatology faculty members and residents representing 80 academic dermatology programs across the country came together to exchange ideas and share success stories for evaluating and selecting URiM candidates for their institution's residency programs. The Intersociety Diversity Task Force partnered with several industry sponsors to help host this workshop.

The goals for the Diversity Champion Workshop were to drive awareness of the role residency programs have in improving diversity of the dermatology workforce, facilitate establishment and development of diversity outreach programs, learn what programs are doing to improve URiM diversity in dermatology, increase awareness of holistic review processes for residency applicants, help expand cultural competence and humility within all residency programs, and contribute to improved patient health outcomes in minority communities. The workshop addressed many topics important to achieve this goal, including mentorship, allyship, holistic residency applicant review, recruitment, and retention.

The AAD has also developed a "Diversity Champion Toolkit" to aid dermatologists in increasing early awareness and exposure of those URiM to dermatology. This toolkit includes ideas for community and faculty dermatologists to establish outreach programs in high schools, colleges, and medical schools in their communities with the goal of reaching students from underserved backgrounds.

Pathway Programs and Mentorship

The AAD has also created the "Pathways: Inclusivity in Dermatology" program in an effort to encourage high school students from black, Latinx, and indigenous communities to pursue dermatology. Through scholarship offerings, skills workshops, mentorship programs, and leadership training, the initiative aims to increase the number of dermatology residents from black, Latinx, and indigenous communities by more than 50% by the year 2027, increase dermatology program faculty from black, Latinx, and indigenous backgrounds by 2%, and increase "Pathways" touchpoints promoting dermatology to black, Latinx, and indigenous high school, college, and medical school students by 10% each year.[7]

The AAD partnered with Nth Dimensions, a US pipeline program for women and minorities seeking to match in competitive medical specialties, which hosts BioSkills workshops in an effort to offer URiM students early exposure opportunities to learn basic dermatologic procedures. These workshops are run in collaboration with Student National Medical Association (SNMA) and Latino Medical Student Association and are hosted at historically black colleges and universities, such as Morehouse School of Medicine, Howard University School of Medicine, and Meharry Medical College, in an effort to reach URiM students. Through partnership with Nth Dimensions, the Academy has sponsored several AAD–Nth Dimension Scholars to participate in an 8-week clinical and research internship with dermatology physicians across the country.

In addition, medical students who are URiM are eligible and encouraged to apply to participate in the AAD Diversity Mentorship Program. This 1-month, full-time, 40-hour per week program consists of hands-on experience in clinical dermatology as well as one-on-one mentorship with a dermatologist. In addition, monetary grants are awarded to students who participate in this program to assist with travel and living expenses. Through this initiative, underrepresented medical students are encouraged to pursue a career in dermatology, ultimately helping to increase diversity in this field.

Improving Health Equity

The AAD has created the AAD Access Derm Program, a philanthropic teledermatology program designed to deliver dermatologic expertise to underserved populations. Through the volunteer efforts of board-certified, AAD member dermatologists and residents, this service has been able to provide free of charge safe and secure consultations to more than 300,000 patients in the United States who would otherwise be unable to access dermatologic care.[8]

AAD has also collaborated with Visual Dx in starting Project IMPACT (Improving Medicine's Power to Address Care and Treatment) in an effort to reduce health disparities and help bring health equity to all people. The goal of this project is to better equip dermatologists to recognize disease presentation in different skin colors in an effort to reduce racial bias in health care.

Awards

In 2021, the AAD created 2 awards to recognize treatment and research of underserved populations. The John Kenney Jr, MD Lifetime Achievement Award was established in honor of Dr John Kenney Jr, the first African American member of the AAD. This $10,000 award recognizes dermatologists who are committed to improving the treatment of patients from underserved populations, including skin of color patients throughout their careers. The A. Paul Kelly, MD Research Award was established to honor of the work of Dr A. Paul Kelly, an expert on skin diseases in people of color and keloidal scarring. This $10,000 award recognizes outstanding dermatologists, who are committed to researching issues associated with skin of color and improving dermatologic care for patients.

Educational Resources

The AAD has established a comprehensive "AAD Diversity Toolkit" with resource guides for health care providers on antiracism, cultural competence, implicit biases, microaggressions, and resources for allyship. A Skin of Color Curriculum Work Group was created in an effort to develop a curriculum to include the diagnosis and effective

treatment of Skin of Color disease and conditions for dermatology residents. This curriculum consists of 60 modules aimed at closing the gap in skin of color education.[8]

WOMEN'S DERMATOLOGIC SOCIETY
Diversity, Equity, and Inclusion Committee

The Women's Dermatologic Society (WDS) task force was created in 2018 to address the low percentage of underrepresented minorities in medicine and dermatology. This task force led to the WDS Diversity, Equity, and Inclusion Committee with the mission to "cultivate diversity, equity, and inclusion within dermatology through the creation of educational experiences, scholarly opportunities, and collegial support." The DEI committee has implemented several initiatives to meet this goal, including establishing a summer research fellowship for URiM students and hosting an annual networking breakfast to connect URiM residents and medical students with faculty members of the WDS. The WDS has also collaborated with the AAD's Intersociety Diversity Task Force to cosponsor initiatives.

Diversity in Leadership

The WDS has successfully included underrepresented women in its leadership structure. The Society elected the first Japanese American WDS president in 2002 and the first black WDS president in 2009 and is the only dermatology organization to have 4 women of color serve in the organization's presidency.[9]

Research and Mentorship

The WDS Student Summer Research Fellowship for URiM students was initiated with the goal of cultivating diverse applicants in the field of dermatology. This grant awards up to $2000 to support participation of a URiM medical student in a full-time 6- to 12-week summer research project under mentorship from a WDS member.[9] The Society has also hosted several networking events for minority students, including an Annual Diversity Breakfast, to provide an opportunity for URiM students across the country to network with resident and dermatologist members of WDS.[9,10]

In addition, the Society has established an Underrepresented in Medicine Resident Research Mentorship Award in an effort to help URiM trainees develop mentoring relationships that might not otherwise be possible owing to distance or funding. This award is open to URiM PGY1, PGY2, or PGY3 dermatology residents and provides up to $2000 for direct expenses for their mentorship experience and research project.

Raising Public Awareness

The WDS has published several articles in the *International Journal of Women's Dermatology (IJWD)* specifically targeted at increasing the number of minority women in dermatology, including "If you want to be it, it helps to see it: Examining the need for diversity in dermatology" and "Turning the Tide: How the Women's Dermatologic Society Leads in Diversifying Dermatology"[9,10] The organization has worked to increase the number of publications related to skin of color in *IJWD*, and as of March 2021, there were 26 publications in the Journal specific to skin and hair of color, as well as diversity and inclusion issues.[9] In addition, the organization has hosted several panel discussions to encourage diversity in dermatology, including "WDS Diversity, Equity, and Inclusion Panel Discussion: The Match Process" and "Why Every Dermatologist Should be Involved in Advocacy."

Partnership

The WDS collaborated with the AAD's Intersociety Diversity Task Force to cosponsor the Diversity Champion Workshop in 2019, and through this initiative has been working toward increasing fellowships and networking opportunities for first-through third-year medical students.

ASSOCIATION OF PROFESSORS OF DERMATOLOGY
Antiracism Statement

In April 2021, the APD published a statement on antiracism in academic medicine stating that "[the APD Residency Program Directors] stand strongly in support of our colleagues in residency and fellowship leadership as well as our trainees who come from diverse backgrounds, especially those from groups historically marginalized in our country."[11] This statement condemned racism and discrimination at all levels of medicine and called for a closer look at diversifying educational and leadership systems. The statement also announced the establishment of a DEI Workgroup within the APD Residency Program Directors Section to create an inclusive group of program leaders with goals to build DEI-related residency curricular elements and resources for faculty development.

Partnerships

The APD has detailed several initiatives to highlight and recognize contributions of trainees of color. These initiatives are geared toward partnerships with other dermatologic organizations, such as participating in mentorship programs for URiM students in association with the NMA Dermatology Section and Dermatology Interest Group Association. The APD has collaborated with the AAD's Intersociety Diversity Task Force to cosponsor initiatives. In addition, the APD Annual Meeting has hosted several sessions on issues related to improving DEI in dermatology.

Residency-Focused Initiatives

The APD has formally recommended implementing practices that elevate and recognize the contributions of colleagues and trainees of color and has stated a goal to promote "increased diversity in dermatology resident recruitment with development of guidelines for holistic review and innovation in the application/selection process to create equitable practices." To this end, the organization has set forth initiatives to address these issues, including the creation of virtual forums for program directors and academic faculty to discuss systemic racism and DEI efforts in dermatology.[12]

SOCIETY FOR INVESTIGATIVE DERMATOLOGY
Diversity, Equity, and Inclusion Committee

The SID diversity and inclusion committee was started as an ad hoc committee in May 2017 and is now a formal committee with a goal to "[i]ncrease diversity and inclusion in the membership and programming activities of the SID."

Diversity in Investigative Dermatology

The SID started the Freinkel Diversity Scholars fellowship program in May 2019 with the goal of increasing diversity in dermatology by recognizing women and underrepresented minorities in SID who are conducting research in dermatology and cutaneous biology and are committed to careers in investigative dermatology.[13] Fellows in this program receive a $7500 grant awarded to their institution for 2 years to support research and travel activities. Women and underrepresented minority applicants who are early in their careers or who are academic faculty engaged in investigative dermatology or cutaneous biology are eligible to apply for this fellowship. The organization also sponsors travel grants for underrepresented minority laboratory technicians, medical/graduate students, residents, fellows, and junior faculty to attend the annual SID conference. In addition, the SID has greatly increased representation of women as speakers in the annual meeting and as members, and from 1998 to 2017, the percentage of female SID members increased from 20% to 40%.[13,14]

Intersociety Collaborations

Through partnership with SNMA, SID members have served as research, clinical, and personal mentors for URiM students interested in dermatology as well as provide shadowing opportunities for these students.[13] The SID has collaborated with the AAD's Intersociety Diversity Task Force to cosponsor initiatives, is specifically working to develop a program to support research "gap" years, and has created an SID member pool for mentoring.

Educational Resources

In 2021, the SID hosted a Diversity and Inclusion Panel Discussion with dermatologists from URiM backgrounds to discuss their personal experiences in medical school, challenges they faced as students from underrepresented backgrounds, what allies can do to support URiM students throughout their training, and how to prevent implicit bias in the medical school and dermatology application process. In addition, the SID Web site hosts a "Diversity and Inclusion Toolkit" page with suggested readings to promote better understanding of diversity and inclusion.

SKIN OF COLOR SOCIETY
Mission

The mission of the SOCS is to promote awareness of and excellence within skin of color dermatology through research, education, mentorship, and advocacy. The Society was built under the core values of equity, excellence, mentorship, research, innovation, and education and has stated a commitment to increasing DEI in dermatology to advance patient care. The Society published a diversity statement denouncing prejudice, discrimination, and systemic racism and speaking out against racial injustice and disparities in health care. The organization has also partnered with brands, pharmaceutical agencies, and sponsors to aid contributions to help fulfill its mission.

Diversity Task Force

At the 2016 Annual Meeting, the SOCS initiated the Diversity in Action Task Force with the goal of building supportive networks and resources to increase numbers of individuals who are underrepresented in dermatology. In addition, the newly created Under-Representation of SOC Images in Dermatology Task Force has recently undertaken the task of systematically diversifying and expanding the representation of skin of color images in dermatology databases. The SOCS has collaborated with the AAD's Intersociety Diversity Task Force to cosponsor initiatives.

Educational Resources

The theme for the 18th Annual Skin of Color Society Scientific Symposium was "Diversity in Action: Science, Healthcare & Society" and featured several panels specific to dermatologic conditions in skin of color, such as keloids, pigmentary disorders, and aesthetics. Outside of the symposium, the SOCS has also hosted virtual lecture series on topics such as "Truths and Myths in Skin Aging and Skin Cancer in Darker Skin Types."

The SOCS Web site features a "Dermatology Resources" page showcasing a list of skin of color textbooks and ethnic skin centers in the United States. In addition, the SOCS has created an "Educational Video Library" with dermatology education articles and video to learn more about skin diseases that impact patients with skin of color. These videos are free and accessible for providers and patients. In addition, the SOCS also runs a blog discussing DEI issues in dermatology. Most recently, the blog commemorated Black History Month 2022, with a focus on black health and wellness.

In addition, in June 2022, the Society established the "Meeting the Challenge Summit: Diversity in Dermatology Clinical Trials." This interactive summit brought together numerous disciplines and sectors to define the scope of underrepresentation of minorities in dermatologic studies, identify the challenges that impede progress in creating a diverse cohort of study participants, develop actionable recommendations to overcome barriers to progress, and disseminate meeting findings via a prominent publication.

Research

The Annual SOCS Scientific Symposium immediately precedes the Annual AAD Meeting and allows dermatologists and scientists the opportunity to present data on diseases associated with individuals with ethnic skin. During the symposium, the SOCS Research Awards are granted to dermatology residents, fellows, or young dermatologists within the first 8 years of postgraduate training.[15] This award provides 3 annual research grants up to $15,000 to promote dermatology research within the field of skin of color. The SOCS Career Development Award, with an award of up to $100,000, recognizes researchers who have investigative focus on inflammatory dermatologic diseases in skin of color in areas where further clinical, translational, and basic research is needed. In addition, the SOCS has offered virtual grant writing Webinars to improve the scope of dermatology investigation and reduce barriers to skin of color research.

Addressing Disparities

To address disparities affecting dermatology trainees, the SOCS hosts an ongoing "Dermatology Diversity Town Hall Series," an open forum opportunity for medical students, residents, and physicians to interact and gain insights into the issues facing URiM dermatology applicants. Topics discussed in this series have included "The Dermatology Residency Application Process," "Addressing Disparities Impacting URiM Medical Students During COVID-19," and "Diversity, Disparities, Dialogue, & Dermatology."

Mentorship

The SOCS offers several mentorship opportunities for dermatology trainees. The SOCS Observership Grant awards $2000 grants to dermatology residents and junior faculty to enable study with an SOCS mentor in an effort to foster academic and research skills that can further their careers as leaders in skin of color dermatology. The SOCS Mentorship Program is a comprehensive program open to medical students and residents that allows mentorship opportunities for young physicians and medical students with an approved SOCS expert.

AMERICAN SOCIETY FOR DERMATOLOGIC SURGERY
Diversity, Equity, and Inclusion Work Group

The ASDS created a DEI value statement that asserts "commitment to non-discrimination, antiracism, inclusion, cultural sensitivity and humility with the goal of advancing health equity for racial and ethnic, minorities, individuals living with disability, and sexual and gender minority people regardless of background." In April 2020, the ASDS created a DEI Work Group with the goal of promoting cultural competency and awareness within dermatology, increasing diversity within ASDS among members, leaders, volunteers, and speakers, and educating URiM trainees about general and procedural dermatology.[12]

The ASDS DEI Work Group developed a DEI position statement supporting the Society's commitment to addressing implicit bias, ensuring nondiscrimination, mitigating health disparities facing minority populations, addressing barriers to health care, increasing sensitivity to the needs and health of black, indigenous, and people of color (BIPOC), LGBTQ+, sexual and gender minority (SGM) individuals, and supporting the recruitment and retention of such individuals and others URiM. This statement also addressed the need for an increase of diversity in the physician workforce inclusive of BIPOC, LGBTQ+, and SGM individuals to ensure that workforce representation reflects the diversity of the US population. The ASDS DEI Work Group has also created a diversity call-to-action video recognizing the need for change and acknowledging and using privilege to aid diverse populations.[12]

Mentorship

The ASDS has addressed the need for an increased pipeline of URiM, LGBTQ+, and SGM students entering medical school, dermatology residency programs, and dermatology fellowships. To meet this goal, the Society created the Rise Up Mentorship Program in an effort to support URiM trainees in dermatology who are looking for guidance and to expand their support network. Through this program, dermatology mentors are paired with mentees from URiM, SGM, and LGBTQ+ backgrounds to share their professional knowledge, skills, and experiences and help mentees make connections and develop leadership acumen.

Ambassador Program

The ASDS created the DEI Ambassador program with the goal of promoting a culture of acceptance and nondiscrimination. Through this program, dermatology practitioners are encouraged to commit to nondiscrimination, antiracism, inclusion, cultural sensitivity, and humility with the goal of advancing health equity for minority populations. Applicants interested in being DEI Ambassadors sign a pledge to commit to the expectations of the role and are encouraged to attend educational programs on DEI and foster intentional dialogues on ways to create more just and equitable environments.

Educational Resources

The ASDS position statement cites a need to institute inclusive curricula in medical education to address the unique health concerns of racial and ethnic minorities as well as LGBTQ+/SGM individuals. To meet this goal, the organization has hosted a series of DEI Webinars, including "Transgender and Gender Diverse Individuals: Considerations in Procedural Dermatology," "Procedural Dermatology and Skin of Color,"

"Addressing Macro- and Micro-Aggressions in the Practice," and "Rethinking Cosmetic Clinical Trials Focusing on Skin of Color." The goal of these Webinars is to tackle key issues facing dermatologic surgery and dermatology from a practice, patient, and forward-facing perspective and facilitating better understanding of these complex issues. The ASDS also hosted a plenary session entitled "Many Faces: Cultural and Ethnic Diversity in Dermatology" at the 2021 ASDS Annual Meeting to promote increased diversity in dermatology.

In addition, the ASDS Web site has links to resources, including a presentation on Diversifying Your Practice and Inner Circle and the AMA STEPS Forward Toolkit "Racial and Health Equity: Concrete STEPS for Health Systems." The Society has also developed a diversity curriculum for the Cosmetic Fellowship Program through the Future Leaders Network, a 1-year curriculum that provides leadership and project management training for ASDS/American Society for Dermatologic Surgery Association (ASDSA) fellows and graduating resident physicians.

Diversity, Equity, and Inclusion Publications

The ASDS is working toward developing a diversity special issue for *Dermatologic Surgery* journal and has established a standing column *Diversifying Dermatology* in *Currents,* the organization's quarterly magazine. The organization is also working with editors of *Dermatologic Surgery* to include safeguards to ensure insensitive content is not being published and has a mission to expand participation of URiM members in the journal.

Partnership

The ASDS is a cosponsor of AAD's Intersociety Diversity Task Force. The ASDS has also advocated for gender-affirming care in partnership with the ASDSA, and through this initiative, members of the ASDS sent letters to all 50 state governors and the mayor of DC, urging them to veto legislation banning gender-affirming medical care for minors.

THE DERMATOLOGY SECTION OF THE NATIONAL MEDICAL ASSOCIATION
Mission

As a subgroup of the larger NMA, a goal of the Dermatology Section of the NMA (NMA Derm) is to increase the number of African Americans and other underrepresented groups in the field of dermatology. In June 2020, in collaboration with the SOCS, the NMA Derm published an editorial entitled "A Time for Resolve, Change, Unity, and Hope," speaking out against racial injustice and detailing the need for increasing the number of dermatologists of skin of color.

Mentorship

The NMA Derm Mentorship Committee was established to increase representation of African Americans and other students of color in dermatology. The goal of this program is to provide one-on-one guidance for URiM medical students on the application and interviewing process as well as research, shadowing, professional development, and mentorship beyond residency training.[16]

In addition, through partnership with Nth Dimensions and as part of the AAD Intersociety Diversity Task Force, NMA Derm members serve as moderators for skills workshops, hosts for the summer intern program, and presenters for the lecture series.

Research

The NMA Derm Research Committee strives to create relevant research experiences for African American patients, medical students, and research investigators. Through this committee, there is support available for research efforts addressing health disparities and disease burdens in African Americans and underserved communities. There are also partnership opportunities available for URiM students seeking opportunities for research, which are designed to improve treatment outcomes and quality of life of African American patients. In addition, in 2021, NMA Derm established a monthly journal club covering topics related to skin of color, hosted by established experts on the disease topic.

In 2005, NMA Derm established the first John A. Kenney, MD Resident and Fellow Research Symposium at the NMA Annual Convention and Scientific Assembly in honor of Dr John Kenney. This symposium has been occurring annually, and medical students, residents, and fellows from URiM groups who are interested in dermatology, dermatopathology, and dermatologic surgery are eligible to participate. In 2016, NMA Derm similarly established the A. Paul Kelly, MD Medical Student Dermatology Symposium as a tribute to Dr Kelly. URiM medical students interested in dermatology are eligible to present their research at this symposium.

SOCIETY FOR PEDIATRIC DERMATOLOGY
Equity, Diversity, and Inclusion Committee

The Society for Pediatric Dermatology (SPD) established an Equity, Diversity, and Inclusion (EDI) Committee in 2020 to underscore the Society's commitment to diversity and inclusion within the organization and health care equity for all patients. This committee provides guidance to SPD by monitoring intraorganizational diversity and inclusion efforts and increasing representation as needed.

Research and Mentorship

The Underrepresented in Medicine Mentorship Award was created in 2022 to support the academic pursuits of historically marginalized individuals with disproportionately low representation in pediatric dermatology. The goal of this award is to expose dermatology residents to the practice of pediatric dermatology, develop mentoring relationships, and recruit URiM physicians into pediatric dermatology.

The SPD has also collaborated with the Pediatric Dermatology Research Alliance to establish a mentor grant for URiM students to perform research and be mentored in pediatric dermatology. In addition, the Society has been highlighting URiM leaders and practicing Pediatric Dermatologists in the "mentoring moments" section of their newsletter.

Diversity, Equity, and Inclusion Publications

The "Equity, Diversity, and Inclusion" special issue of *Pediatric Dermatology* was published in November 2021 with the goal of highlighting topics, including issues pertaining to skin of color, LGBTQIA+ populations, and patients with physical/intellectual disability.[17] This issue addressed many different historically marginalized populations based on race, ethnicity, income, disability status, gender identification, and sexual orientation.

Educational Resources

The SPD has established an initiative to include a DEI lecture at each of their annual meetings and is working toward establishing a networking breakfast at the annual meeting for URiM attendings and trainees.

In addition, the Society has created several diversity-focused patient perspectives handouts, including "More Than Skin Deep: Impact of Skin Disease and Visible Differences on a Child's Mental and Social Well-Being" and "Curly and Coily Hair Care," discussing differences in black/African American hair and skin and how to talk about visible differences. These handouts also include special recommendations for various populations, such as special considerations for patients with Down syndrome and transgender youth. All handouts have an option for Spanish translations to maximize access.

Members of the SPD have also given several lectures on DEI topics, including "Achieving Racial Equality in Dermatology Care" and "Detailing Racial Disparities in Dermatology at Health Care Crossroad."

In May 2021, in light of violence occurring against Asian Americans in the United States, the SPD recognized Asian American and Pacific Islander Heritage Month and condemned violent acts and hate speech against Asian Americans. In addition, the SPD posted a list of antiracist resources, including readings, toolkits, and trainings, to support the Asian American Community.

SUMMARY

Recent trends in DEI initiatives across US dermatology organizations include creation of DEI-specific committees, funding for URiM students to pursue skin of color research, and tailored mentorship for URiM students. Along with increased dialogue on expanding diversity in dermatology resident recruitment, upstream efforts have also been implemented to encourage high school– and college-aged students to pursue the field of dermatology. The most prominent DEI successes have been collaborations between dermatology organizations to host large-scale events, such as the Diversity Champion Workshop, to further discourse on recruiting minority trainees.

These collective efforts by dermatology organizations to increase the number of minority dermatologists have improved access to the field of dermatology for URiM trainees. However, there is still further work to be done in ensuring adequate representation of minority dermatologists. It is imperative that dermatology organizations continue to expand on their DEI infrastructure, with a focus on interorganization collaboration and pipeline programs.

CLINICS CARE POINTS

- Understanding and increasing the diversity of dermatology providers is a crucial step towards increasing equity.
- Increasing the presence of underrepresented in medicine (URiM) dermatologists helps create a healthcare system that is reflective of the patients it serves.
- It is imperative that dermatologists focus on inclusion of Diversity, Equity, and Inclusion (DEI) initatives when treating their patients and building their practices.

REFERENCES

1. Pandya AG, Alexis AF, Berger TG, et al. Increasing racial and ethnic diversity in dermatology: a call to action. J Am Acad Dermatol 2016;74(3):584–7.

2. Downie J. Diversity in the dermatology workforce: what can we do? Practical Dermatology 2019; 16(7):45–8.

3. Colby SL, Jennifer JO. Projections of the size and composition of the U.S. population: 2014 to 2060. Washington, DC: US Census Bureau; 2015.

4. "AAD Strategic Plan." *American Academy of Dermatology*, Available at: https://assets.ctfassets. net/1ny4yoiyrqia/1nLd2vP2SprOhJsMTVjNY4/ 869245873b9ecf5a67721bba842b3958/strategic_ plan.pdf

5. Diversity in Dermatology: Diversity Committee Approved Plan 2021-2023. American Academy of Dermatology 2021;. https://assets.ctfassets.net/ 1ny4yoiyrqia/xQgnCE6ji5skUlcZQHS2b/ 65f0a9072811e11afcc33d043e02cd4d/DEI_Plan. pdf.

6. Position Statement on Dermaology Workforce Diversity and Health Disparities. American Academy of Dermatology 2021;. https://server.aad.org/Forms/ Policies/Uploads/PS/PS-Dermatology%20Workforce %20Diversity%20and%20Health%20Disparities.pdf.

7. Pathways: inclusivity in dermatology. American Academy of Dermatology. https://www.aad.org/member/ career/diversity/diversity-pathways#:~:text=The% 20Pathways%20program%20is%20working,and% 20interest%20to%20pursue%20a. [Accessed 14 October 2022].

8. Lester JC, Taylor SC. Two pandemics: opportunities for diversity, equity and inclusion in dermatology. Int J Womens Dermatol 2021;7(2):137–8.

9. Sekyere NAN, Grimes PE, Roberts WE, et al. Turning the tide: how the women's dermatologic society leads in diversifying dermatology. Int J Womens Dermatol 2020;7(2):135–6.

10. Perez V, Gohara M. If you want to be it, it helps to see it: examining the need for diversity in dermatology. Int J Womens Dermatol 2020;6(3):206–8.

11. APD Residency Program Directors Section Statement on Anti-Racism in Academic Medicine. Association of Professors of Dermatology 2021;. https:// www.dermatologyprofessors.org/files/Anti-racism% 20and%20anti-discrimination%20statement.pdf.

12. Desai SR, Khanna R, Glass D, et al. Embracing diversity in dermatology: creation of a culture of equity and inclusion in dermatology. Int J Womens Dermatol 2021;7(4):378–82.

13. Horsley V, Glass D, Minnillo R, et al. Diversity is excellence: initiatives in the society for investigative dermatology to broaden participation. J Invest Dermatol 2019;139(10):2217–9.

14. Swerlick RA. Diversity and inclusion: the right initiative and a smart initiative for the society for investigative dermatology. J Invest Dermatol 2018;138(9): 1887–9.

15. Subash J, Tull R, McMichael A. Diversity in dermatology: a society devoted to skin of color. Cutis 2017;99(5):322–4.

16. Massick S. Fueling the pipeline: dermatology mentorship for underrepresented minority students. Women's Dermatologic Society 2021;. https://www. womensderm.org/UserFiles/file/Publications/ Editorials/22_UIMMentorship_Massick_ CORRECTED.pdf.

17. Benjamin L, Gupta D, Pourciau CY. An introduction to the equity, diversity and inclusion supplemental issue of pediatric dermatology: a message from the guest editors. Pediatr Dermatol 2021;38(Suppl 2):1.

Steps Leaders Can Take to Increase Diversity, Enhance Inclusion, and Achieve Equity

Henry W. Lim, MD

KEYWORDS

- Diversity • Equity and inclusion • LGBTQ/sexual and gender minority • Holistic review • Gender

KEY POINTS

- Since the importance of skin of color (SOC) and diversity, equity, and inclusion (DEI) was recognized in the late 1990s, due to the advocacy and effort of several highly visible leaders in dermatology, noticeable progress has been achieved. These progresses include increased commitment by the American Academy of Dermatology (AAD) and other societies to promote DEI and increased number of underrepresented in medicine entering dermatology residency.
- Greater than 60% of dermatology residents are women. Effort needs to be made to increase the representation of women in senior dermatology leadership positions.
- The AAD Expert Resource Group on LGBTQ/Sexual and Gender Minority Health has been active in establishing dermatology module, webinars, mentorship, and other activities. This effort needs to be continued and supported.
- Commitment by highly visible leaders, engagement of other societies and leaders of the academic departments, inclusivity in DEI to include gender and sexual orientation, and cultivation of allies and allyship are important steps to be taken for successful implementation of DEI.

In this chapter, steps taken by leaders (**Box 1**) in dermatology to improve diversity, equity, and inclusion (DEI), which started in the late 1990s, are described, and progress made to date is highlighted. Based on the efforts made by dermatology leaders, valuable lessons learned are summarized.

DIVERSITY, EQUITY, AND INCLUSION IN DERMATOLOGY

The importance of recognition of diseases in individuals with skin of color (SOC) was best highlighted by the establishment of Skin of Color Center at St Luke-Roosevelt's Hospital in New York City by Susan Taylor, MD, in 1999. This was followed by establishments of several centers in dermatology departments in the United States;

by 2020, there were 15 such centers.[1] These centers focused on the dermatologic care of diseases commonly seen in individuals with SOC, education of dermatologists and trainees on many unique manifestations of these diseases, and conducting and promoting research in SOC.

The aforementioned was followed by the founding of Skin of Color Society (SOCS) in 2014, again by Susan Taylor, MD (**Fig. 1**). SOCS is now the major society that focuses on advancing research in SOC, as well as a venue for mentoring the next generation of dermatologists who are interested in this important aspect of dermatology. Starting from 2000s, several textbooks on SOC have been published, and continuing medical education sessions on SOC topics also started to be offered,

Department of Dermatology, Henry Ford Health, New Center One, 3031 West Grand Boulevard, Suite 800, Detroit, MI 48202, USA
E-mail address: hlim1@hfhs.org

Dermatol Clin 41 (2023) 371–375
https://doi.org/10.1016/j.det.2022.10.009
0733-8635/23/© 2022 Elsevier Inc. All rights reserved.

> **Box 1**
> **Important steps to be taken by leaders to achieve diversity, equity, and inclusion**
>
> 1. Commitment by and continued engagement of highly visible leaders.
> 2. Engagement of other societies in dermatology.
> 3. Engagement of dermatology department leaders and educators.
> 4. Education and engagement of the next generation of dermatologists.
> 5. Inclusivity in DEI to include gender and sexual orientation.
> 6. Cultivation of allies and allyship.

including at the annual meetings of the American Academy of Dermatology (AAD).

As a better understanding of dermatology in SOC occurred, it was increasingly clear that further progress can only be made by increasing the diversity of dermatology care givers. It is known, for example, some patients perceived that they received better quality of care in a race-concordant visit. Black patients with hair problems would be more comfortable to be treated by care providers who demonstrate good knowledge and familiarity of their hair care practice. Understanding of and sensitivity to the unique cultural practice of female patients who are fully clothed from head to toe is an important aspect of care of these patients. Data from Association of American Medical Colleges shows that physicians from underrepresented in medicine (URM) background

have a higher likelihood of practicing in underserved areas,[2] which helps to address the health care disparity seen in the United States.

As discussed elsewhere in this issue, dermatology is the second least diverse specialty in medicine. The importance of DEI was highlighted by Bruce Wintroub, MD, then vice dean and chair of dermatology at University of California, San Francisco. Dr Wintroub presented this topic in Clarence S. Livingood, MD, lecture at the plenary session of the annual meeting of AAD in 2015; this was followed by a call-to-action article to increase racial and ethnic diversity in dermatology.[3]

In March 2017, Henry W. Lim, MD started his term as president of the AAD. In his inaugural address, he emphasized that effort should be made so that "the face of Dermatology would reflect the face of our patients." To initiate the steps to achieve this goal, an AAD President's Conference on Diversity was held in August 2017. Although AAD is the nation's largest dermatology organization, it was recognized that such an effort required the engagement of other dermatologic societies. The conference was sponsored not only by the AAD but also by Association of Professors of Dermatology (APD), Society for Investigative Dermatology (SID), and American Dermatological Association (ADA). Recommendations from the conference included the following: (1) to increase pipeline/pathway of URM to medical school; (2) to increase the interest of URM medical students in dermatology; and (3) to increase the number of URM in dermatology residency.[4]

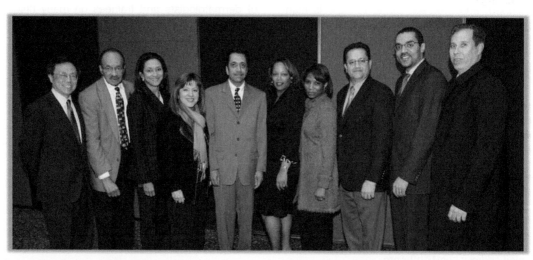

Fig. 1. Skin of color society. Founder, Susan Taylor, MD (third from left) and some of the founding members of the Board of Directors (2004).

Action steps taken following the conference included the following:

- The presence of dermatology booth at the national meetings of Student National Medical Association and Latino Medical Student Association, jointly sponsored by AAD and other dermatology societies; this was precedent setting, as Dermatology had not had official booth at these meetings. These booths were jointly sponsored by AAD and other dermatologic societies.
- Establishment of annual Diversity Champion Workshop. The workshop was organized by inviting all academic dermatology departments to send representatives ("champions") to discuss steps that can be done within each department, such as informal reception for URM medical students ("pizza party," initiated by Amit Pandya, MD, University of Texas Southwestern Medical Center, an early proponent of DEI), mentorship, outreach to medical schools, formation of departmental DEI committee, and so forth.
- Continued encouragement on engagement by other societies in dermatology, which include APD, SID, SOCS, and Women's Dermatologic Society (WDS).

In subsequent meetings of Diversity Champion Workshop, as well as in meetings of APD, holistic review of residency applicants was discussed.[5] Although this had already taken place in a few departments, more in-depth discussion took place. In holistic review, rather than focusing exclusively on academic performance, distance traveled, life experience, and resilience of the candidates were taken into consideration. Faculty selection committee members were encouraged to take implicit bias test and training.

In addition to race and ethnicity, gender and sexual orientation are also integral part of DEI. Women have had strong representation in dermatology residency programs, ranging from 58% to 68% for graduating class of 2017 to 2024 (Table 1). Although data on senior dermatology academic leaders (full professors or chairs) are not readily available, data from US medical schools showed differences between men and women faculty (Table 2).[6] Based on data from 2020, 27% of men faculty in US medical schools were full professors and 2.5% were chairs. Corresponding percentages for women faculty were 13% and 0.9%, respectively. It is likely that similar trend is also seen in dermatology. Clearly, more effort needs to be done in correcting this inequity.

Recognizing that sexual orientation and gender identity need to be addressed in discussion on

Table 1
Percentage of women residents in dermatology

Residency Completion Year	Cohort n	Median Age	Female (%)	Male (%)
2017	336	31	64	36
2018	364	31	68	32
2019	374	31	65	35
2020	379	31	61	39
2021	450	31	58	42
2022	532	32	58	42
2023	530	31	61	39
2024	494	31	62	38

Data provided by the American Academy of Dermatology, May 2022. Used with permission.

DEI, an AAD Expert Resource Group (ERG) on lesbian, gay, bisexual, transgender, and queer (LGBTQ)/sexual and gender minority (SGM) health was established during the AAD presidency of Henry Lim, MD. Activity done by this ERG has included LGBTQ/SGM dermatology module, webinars, mentorship, and active involvement by its members in various AAD committees and task forces.

Early measurable improvements have been observed (Box 2). Many dermatology departments now have DEI committee, and holistic review is more commonly practiced in residency selection process. Many departments now provide stipends for rotators with financial needs; most of them are URMs. Mentorships for URMs are offered by many dermatologic organizations. In August 2020, the AAD Board of Directors formally recognized that increased focus on DEI needed to be done at all levels of the organization. An AAD Intersociety Diversity Task Force has been established, becoming a part of the organization structure of the ADD. Members of this Task Force consist of not only appointees by the AAD but also representatives of other dermatologic organizations, thus

Table 2
Gender distribution among US medical school faculty

	Women		Men	
Full-time faculty	79,174	—	105,307	—
Full professors	10,421	13%	28,544	27%
Chairs	696	0.9%	2,602	2.5%

Data from Choi AMK, Rustgi AK. Diversity in Leadership at Academic Medical Centers: Addressing Underrepresentation Among Asian American Faculty. JAMA. 2021;326(7):605-606.

> **Box 2**
> **Summary of accomplishments in dermatology**
>
> Increased focus on DEI throughout the AAD structure
>
> DEI committee in many dermatologic societies and academic departments
>
> AAD Expert Resource Group (ERG) on lesbian, gay, bisexual, transgender, and queer (LGBTQ)/sexual and gender minority (SGM) health
>
> Holistic review of residency applicants
>
> Mentorship for URMs
>
> Stipend for rotators with financial needs
>
> AAD Intersociety Diversity Task Force
>
> AAD SOC curriculum
>
> AAD Curriculum for Advancing Racial Equity
>
> DEI symposium at AAD annual meeting
>
> Increased percentage of diversity-focused sessions at AAD
>
> Increased percentage of URM in dermatology residency

providing an opportunity for continued interactions of all dermatologic organizations in addressing DEI. An AAD Skin of Color curriculum has been established, and Curriculum for Advancing Racial Equity (CARE) is being rolled out. The first AAD DEI symposium was included in the program of AAD annual meeting, starting in 2022. The plenary session of the 2022 annual meeting included 2 lectures on DEI topics. Diversity-focused sessions at annual meetings of AAD had increased from 2.5% in 2013 to 6.8% in 2019.[7] As importantly, the percentage of Hispanic/Latino dermatology residents has increased from 3.1% in 2017 to 4.0% in 2021 and Black, 3.5% to 4.8% (**Table 3**).[8] Because of the small number, unfortunately, similar data could not be generated for American Indian, Alaska Native, Native Hawaiian, and Pacific Islanders. In 2021, there were 450 residents who completed dermatology training in the United States; the March 2022 match data showed that at least 52 URM had matched into dermatology.

Leadership Lessons Learned

The collective experience of leaders in dermatology in advancing DEI has provided valuable insights, which can be summarized as follows (see **Table 3**):

1. Commitment by and continued engagement of highly visible leaders. As in medicine in general, DEI was a relatively new concept in dermatology when the topic started to be discussed in the late 1990s. DEI was introduced by several highly visible and committed leaders of the specialty. The continuous engagement of leaders in many levels of dermatology organizations to transform the culture and to infuse DEI concept into the core value of the organization was essential to the success of the effort.

2. Engagement of other societies in dermatology. Although AAD is the largest dermatologic organization in the United States, for DEI to be successful, the engagement of other societies is essential. From the initiation of this effort, key societies are included in DEI initiatives of the AAD; this resulted in DEI sessions and committees in those societies, and as a consequence, their members are informed and educated on the relevance and importance of DEI in our specialty.

3. Engagement of dermatology department leaders and educators. Members of the Association of Professors of Dermatology (APD) are dermatology chairs and residency program directors; it is therefore essential that they have a good understanding of DEI, as they determine the future workforce in our specialty. APD was a participant of the first AAD initiative, the 2017 President's Conference on Diversity. APD has consistently been the cosponsor of the annual Diversity Champion Workshop, resulting in familiarity in many dermatology departments with DEI, and this facilitated the implementation of holistic review of residency candidates, administration of implicit bias training of the faculty, and formation of DEI committee in many departments.

4. Education and engagement of the next generation of dermatologists. Young dermatologists are the future of our specialty. In order for DEI to continue to be an integral part of dermatology, awareness, education, and engagement of young and upcoming leaders in dermatology is essential. Within the AAD, intentional efforts have been made to have the next generation of leaders to lead many of the DEI committees, Diversity Champion Workshop, and other DEI-focused activities; mentorship was provided as appropriate.

5. Inclusivity in DEI. In addition to race and ethnicity, other relevant aspects of DEI in dermatology include gender and sexual orientation. Although women represent 60% of dermatology residents, similar to house of medicine in general, there is still a sizable gap between percentage of women in senior leadership levels compared to men. Although the reasons are multifactorial, continued effort needs to make by all on sponsorship and

Table 3
Racial/ethnic distribution of dermatology residents

Res.Grad. Year	Total Active	White (%)	Asian (%)	Hispanic/ Latino (%)	Black/African American (%)	Multiple Races/ Ethnicities (New in 2021) (%)	Other (%)	Unknown (%)
2017	1424	57.7	13.7	3.1	3.5	—	3.6	18.3
2018	1517	58.2	14.6	2.8	3.0	—	4.5	16.8
2019	1563	56.0	16.0	2.9	3.3	—	5.7	16.0
2020	1594	57.7	17.3	3.8	3.9	—	6.4	10.7
2021	1612	58.1	21.7	4.0	4.8	7.0	2.5	1.6
2019 MED SCHOOL GRADS		54.6	21.6	5.3	6.2	8.0	3.8	.6
2018 DERM WORKFORCE		66.0	12.0	4.4	3.4	.7	1.2	11.9

Data from ACGME Graduate Education Data. Available at: https://www.acgme.org/about-us/publications-and-resources/graduate-medical-education-data-resource-book/). Compiled and provided by courtesy of the American Academy of Dermatology. Accessed May 1, 2022.

mentorship of women in dermatology to achieve equity. Excellent progress made by AAD LGBTQ/SGM Health ERG needs to continue to be supported and promoted.

6. Cultivation of allies and allyship. Allies are individuals who understand and act on the need for the equal and fair treatment of people different than them. Diversity Champion Workshop, for example, strongly promotes allyship, which is an essential factor for the success of DEI initiatives.

In conclusion, because of the effort of many, progress on DEI in dermatology has been made. However, continued effort and engagement by all is needed for the benefit of our specialty and the patients we serve.

DISCLOSURE

H.W. Lim is the vice chair of the Diversity, Equity, Inclusion, and Justice Committee of Henry Ford Health-Michigan State University. No other conflict to disclose.

REFERENCES

1. Tull RZ, Kerby E, Subash JJ, et al. Ethnic skin centers in the United States: Where are we in 2020? J Am Acad Dermatol 2020;83(6):1757–9. Epub 2020 Mar 30. PMID: 32240672.

2. https://www.aamc.org/data-reports/workforce/interactive-data/figure-11-percentage-us-medical-school-matriculants-planning-practice-underserved-area-race. Accessed April 29, 2022

3. Pandya AG, Alexis AF, Berger TG, et al. Increasing racial and ethnic diversity in dermatology: A call to action. J Am Acad Dermatol 2016 Mar;74(3):584–7. Epub 2016 Jan 8. PMID: 26774427.

4. Pritchett EN, Pandya AG, Ferguson NN, et al. Diversity in dermatology: roadmap for improvement. J Am Acad Dermatol 2018;79(2):337–41. Epub 2018 Apr 10. PMID: 29653209.

5. Luke J, Cornelius L, Lim HW. Dermatology resident selection: shifting toward holistic review? J Am Acad Dermatol 2021;84(4):1208–9. Epub 2020 Nov 24. PMID: 33245933.

6. Choi AMK, Rustgi AK. Diversity in leadership at academic medical centers: addressing underrepresentation among Asian American faculty. JAMA 2021; 326(7):605–6.

7. Seale L, Awosika O, Lim HW. Trends in sessions in diversity at the American Academy of Dermatology Annual Meetings: 2013-2019. Int J Womens Dermatol 2021;7(2):197–8.

8. ACGME Graduate Education Data. Compiled and provided by courtesy of the American Academy of Dermatology. 2022. https://www.acgme.org/about-us/publications-and-resources/graduate-medical-education-data-resource-book/. Accessed 29 April 2022.

Moving?

Make sure your subscription moves with you!

To notify us of your new address, find your **Clinics Account Number** (located on your mailing label above your name), and contact customer service at:

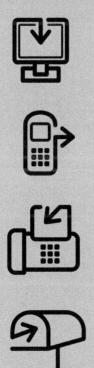

Email: journalscustomerservice-usa@elsevier.com

800-654-2452 (subscribers in the U.S. & Canada)
314-447-8871 (subscribers outside of the U.S. & Canada)

Fax number: 314-447-8029

Elsevier Health Sciences Division
Subscription Customer Service
3251 Riverport Lane
Maryland Heights, MO 63043

Printed and bound by CPI Group (UK) Ltd, Croydon, CR0 4YY

08/05/2025

01864717-0008